AIDS: The Facts

Books by John Langone

DEATH IS A NOUN
A View of the End of Life

GOODBYE TO BEDLAM
Understanding Mental Illness and Retardation

VITAL SIGNS
The Way We Die in America

LIFE AT THE BOTTOM
The People of Antarctica

BOMBED, BUZZED, SMASHED, OR . . . SOBER
A Book about Alcohol

HUMAN ENGINEERING
Marvel or Menace?

LONG LIFE
What We Know and Are Learning about the Aging Process

LIKE, LOVE, LUST
A View of Sex and Sexuality

THORNY ISSUES
How Ethics and Morality Affect the Way We Live

VIOLENCE!
Our Fastest-Growing Public Health Problem

DEAD END
A Book about Suicide

WOMEN WHO DRINK

CHIROPRACTORS
A Consumer's Guide

AIDS: THE FACTS

AIDS: The Facts

JOHN LANGONE

LITTLE, BROWN AND COMPANY
BOSTON   TORONTO

COPYRIGHT © 1988 BY JOHN LANGONE

ALL RIGHTS RESERVED. NO PART OF THIS BOOK MAY BE REPRODUCED
IN ANY FORM OR BY ANY ELECTRONIC OR MECHANICAL MEANS,
INCLUDING INFORMATION STORAGE AND RETRIEVAL SYSTEMS,
WITHOUT PERMISSION IN WRITING FROM THE PUBLISHER, EXCEPT
BY A REVIEWER WHO MAY QUOTE BRIEF PASSAGES IN A REVIEW.

FIRST EDITION

Portions of this book originally appeared
in *Discover* magazine.

Library of Congress Cataloging-in-Publication Data

Langone, John, 1929–
    AIDS: the facts.

    Bibliography: p.
    1. AIDS (Disease)   I. Title.   [DNLM: 1. Acquired
Immunodeficiency Syndrome — popular works.
WD 308 L284a]
RC607.A26L36   1988   616.97′92   87-29309
ISBN 0-316-51413-6
ISBN 0-316-51412-8 (pb)

HC: 10 9 8 7 6 5 4 3 2 1
PB: 10 9 8 7 6 5 4 3 2 1

RRD VA

Published simultaneously in Canada
by Little, Brown & Company (Canada) Limited

PRINTED IN THE UNITED STATES OF AMERICA

For Sana Siwolop and Sally Dorst

Contents

AIDS: The Facts

Premise

To begin with, there was this strange fact; though the infection was there, the moon had often four times circled the earth before clear symptoms of the disease appeared. For when it has once been received into the body it does not immediately declare itself; rather it lies dormant for a certain time and gradually gains strength as it feeds. Meanwhile, however, the sufferers, weighed down by strange heaviness and irresistible languor, are going through life with increasing weakness, moving sluggishly in every limb. Their eyes, too, have lost their natural keenness; the colour is driven from their faces and deserts their unhappy brows.

> — *Girolamo Fracastoro,*
> Syphilis or the French Disease

THE WORDS OF GIROLAMO FRACASTORO — the sixteenth-century Veronese poet-physician whose fame rests upon the Latin verses of his celebrated *Syphilis sive Morbus Gallicus,* a combined mythological and scientific work that gave the venereal disease its name — apply, in some respects, to AIDS, the chilling buzz-acronym of the 1980s.

AIDS is not, of course, syphilis, nor gonorrhea, nor herpes — indeed, it is quite unlike anything else, venereal or otherwise, that virologists and clinicians have ever seen before. AIDS, for "acquired immune deficiency syndrome," is a lethal clinical condition characterized by a breakdown in the body's natural defenses against disease; this immune collapse leaves the way open to a variety of serious illnesses — opportunistic infections — that are not usually found in people with healthy immune systems or that, if they are present under normal circumstances, have only relatively mild repercussions. When they are present in AIDS, they kill.

Still, Fracastoro's words seem eerily apropos. AIDS is, among other things, a venereal disease — that is, one that can be transmitted sexually. The virus that causes it "does not immediately declare itself" but lies dormant for months or years before something as yet unknown, some mechanism still unclear, touches it off and enables it to start up the insidious process that debilitates its victims, enfeebling them to such an extent that they are prey to the life-threatening infections, and to neurological disorders and malignancies as well. And, as in Fracastoro's treatment of his venereal subject, a mythology swirls around AIDS, spinning off a good deal of information that is unfactual, unbelievable, and grossly exaggerated.

At this writing, AIDS — which is correctly defined as the end stage of infection with the AIDS virus and is not a disease that results automatically whenever someone is exposed to the virus — has stricken at least 42,000 Americans since it first surfaced here in 1981 among young, previously healthy homosexual men. It has already killed more than 25,000 of these people, and, because there is as yet no cure, will eventually kill most of the rest, probably within three years. There have been no remissions; there is no vaccine to prevent it.

Despite seemingly authoritative statistics and projections, no one knows exactly how fast the disease is spreading, or precisely how many of those infected with the virus will contract AIDS or its lesser form, ARC (AIDS-related complex). Nor do researchers know why some people progress from ARC to AIDS; for although they suspect a range of predisposing cofactors — such things as a previously weakened immune system, certain infections, recreational intravenous-drug use, to name a few — they cannot yet explain the role or roles these may play. Nor do they even know for certain how the AIDS virus kills the cells it infects, nor even the full range of the cells it prefers. Unanswered questions abound about AIDS at this point — many more, in fact, than have been answered.

With the lack of answers have come myths and misconceptions, some spawned by the moralists among us, some simply by those who are fearful. The disease is divine retribution, we hear, a plague inflicted on gays and drug abusers, the price for unnatural sex and despicable addiction. It is a modern-day Black Death; a wraithlike affliction that threatens everyone in its path; a scourge as easily transmitted as the flu, as inexplicable as a pestilence from another galaxy. There are demands for quarantine, and for mandatory AIDS screening of job applicants, of aliens who would immigrate to the United States, and of Americans who travel abroad.

There is widespread overstatement, too. Some of it is even generated by research institutions that, though they may not deliberately try to mislead an already anxious public, are not averse to employing the new rhetoric of AIDS — which invokes specters of global peril and biological apocalypse — in order to obtain necessary funding and perhaps even to strengthen some researchers' images as AIDS experts, the rescuers in the latest public health crisis.

It is, thus, not easy to keep AIDS in proper perspective. It is even more difficult to chronicle the disease in a book like this one, which involves a writing deadline and has a firm publication date. Such elements, while necessary for the most practical of reasons, unfortunately fix the subject, stopping it in its tracks for the reader and implying that this is all there will be to say and to know about AIDS. Nothing could be further from the truth.

AIDS is a topic in motion, a subject difficult to keep up with and propelled along as much by an unrelenting media and public-agency blitz as by the momentum of the virus itself, which fast outruns the deluge of new research reports and updates that appear weekly in the scientific journals and are presented at the same feverish pace at symposia here and abroad. The virus mutates from one day to the next, thwarting the latest attempts to develop a vaccine; new genes common to all the variants turn up like clockwork (from three, to five, to six, to eight at last count); the current morbidity and mortality figures must be read with dispatch, for they are soon out-of-date; a promising drug works in the test tube, flashes into the headlines, and then is gone and forgotten when it flunks in chimps; one group of researchers turns up evidence showing that the virus causes disease only in previously sick individuals, another team dashes cold water on the data.

Because of such uncertainties, this book is sprinkled — sometimes maddeningly so for writer and reader alike — with maybes, perhapses, possiblys, likelys, and unlikelys. It would be foolhardy to avoid such qualifiers, for AIDS is still an "on-the-other-hand" kind of story, one being spun out by researchers who are often on opposite sides of the fence and who are painfully aware that there is a difference between accumulating facts and promulgating doctrine. It is, thus, still too early to make many definitive statements about AIDS, especially with regard to the behavior of the virus and the disease's future course.

This does not mean, however, that one can only speculate. For despite all the ambiguity, there is still enough solid scientific and epidemiological information to enable one — I speak here for myself — to arrive at some reasonable conclusions about AIDS, conclusions that are repeated several times throughout this book. Chief among them are the following:

- The AIDS virus is not spread casually.
- AIDS is nowhere near the "heterosexual threat" that some have made it out to be — that is, it is not a disease transmitted easily through conventional heterosexual intercourse — nor is it likely to become one soon.
- AIDS in the United States, and in most of the world except Africa, will continue to strike hardest at the risk groups it now afflicts most commonly: homosexual males who engage in anal sex and drug abusers who share needles. (In Africa, where the disease has spread equally among men and women, conditions and practices are so different that they make any comparison to the U.S. outbreak both absurd and irresponsible.)

With a breaking story like this one, the proof of these conclusions will come only with time. Each could eventually be proven wrong (although I firmly doubt that any of them will), and I am prepared to accept the contradictory evidence if that should happen, with my only defense being that when my conclusions were arrived at, they were based on the best data available at the time.

— JOHN LANGONE
October 1987

1

What Is AIDS?

IT IS WELL TO REMEMBER that AIDS is actually the final stage, the most severe end stage, of infection with what we know as the AIDS virus. AIDS is also generally accepted as a syndrome, a collection of specific, life-threatening opportunistic infections and symptoms that is the result of an underlying immune deficiency — a deficiency not caused by any known conditions and illnesses other than infection with the AIDS virus.

The acquired immune deficiency itself — the "AID" part of AIDS — does not kill. It destroys the body's capacity to ward off bacteria and viruses that would ordinarily be fought off by a properly functioning immune system, and it is the diseases, the opportunistic infections, caused by these outside agents that eventually kill the victim; or, death results from a form of cancer, Kaposi's sarcoma, that is far more aggressive in AIDS patients than among those who do not suffer from AIDS. Thus, one can say that AIDS killed the person, since the addition of the "S" defines a syndrome: the collection of diseases and symptoms that resulted from the weakened immune system. Putting it another way, one can say that the AIDS virus itself does not kill, nor does it generally cause the various diseases associated with the syndrome; most of the disastrous events are simply the result of the damage to the immune system. Nor does infection with the virus mean that a person has AIDS or that he or she will get AIDS. It means that the virus has gained entry into that person's body, and that there is a 20- to 50-percent chance —

some say 75-percent — that the infection will advance to AIDS itself.

Unfortunately, however, the acronym AIDS has been used carelessly by the public to describe anything connected with infection by the virus. Thus one hears, "So-and-so has AIDS," when what may really be meant is that the results came out positive on the person's antibody test (a blood test for a factor that may indicate the presence of the AIDS virus), or that the person has one of the non-life-threatening conditions that are associated with some stage between infection and AIDS itself. "If you can write this story without generally referring to this infection as AIDS," one researcher told me, "you'd be performing a service."

2

What Are the Symptoms?

No one can yet say exactly how many of those who carry the
AIDS virus will pass from the initial infected stage to the intermediate stage known as AIDS-related complex (ARC), or
how many ARC patients will go on to develop full-blown AIDS.
But here is a rundown of the signs, symptoms, and diseases that
precede and encompass AIDS.

INFECTION

The initial exposure represents the broad base of the iceberg.
In this category, it is believed, are some 1.5 million Americans,
most of whom are sexually active homosexual and bisexual males,
and men and women who abuse intravenous drugs. A small
percentage of the infected population have received transfused
blood tainted with the AIDS virus, are the heterosexual partners
of someone with AIDS, are infants born to infected mothers,
or are unclassified (though most likely these are undetected
members of one of the other high-risk groups).

Generally, members of the infected group show laboratory
evidence of infection — that is, antibodies to the virus are seen
in their blood samples — but no symptoms, although a short-
term, mononucleosislike disorder, with swollen glands, is occasionally present. (Antibodies are proteins that the body raises
in response to an infection.) People in this classification are
presumably capable of passing the virus along if they engage in

high-risk behavior such as being the active, insertive partner in anal intercourse or the steady heterosexual partner of an uninfected individual, or if they share needles. A seemingly healthy mother, too, may pass the infection along to her infant, before, during, or after birth (through breast-feeding).

Current estimates suggest that an infected person who is without symptoms will probably develop detectable antibodies to the virus two to eight weeks after the initial exposure, but in some cases six or more months may pass before there is such evidence of infection. But while the time that elapses between infection and the presence of antibodies may be charted, the length of time that an infected individual will remain free of symptoms seems to vary widely, from days or weeks to many years, depending on how the infection was acquired. When symptoms do appear, the individual falls into the next category: AIDS-related complex.

AIDS-RELATED COMPLEX (ARC)

This more severe, intermediate stage of an AIDS-virus infection has gone by various names: AIDS-prodrome, pre-AIDS, lesser AIDS, lymphadenopathy syndrome. There are no reliable data on how many people who test positive to the AIDS virus will move into this category (one early estimate was 25 percent), nor, as was mentioned earlier, what cofactors, if any, will play a part in that progression or in moving the infection along to AIDS itself.

The ARC category is ill-defined (in fact, there is no nationally accepted definition of it) and somewhat controversial, since many of its ever-growing range of symptoms and illnesses are also found in patients who meet the technical definition of AIDS itself; often the difference may well be semantic. A number of physicians and researchers, in fact, favor scrapping the ARC category altogether and putting it under AIDS — a move that has the backing of ARC patients who feel they are unfairly denied the social services and disability benefits allowed AIDS patients. (At this writing, the CDC — the Centers for Disease Control, the sprawling agency in Atlanta where the government's disease detectives are based — had proposed to state health officials that they add the most severe forms of ARC, as well as irreversible neurological disorders, to the list of AIDS cases.) Estimates as to how many Americans have ARC are fairly unreliable, but 170,000 is a generally accepted figure.

Generally speaking, the symptoms and the ailments that often appear under the ARC heading vary in severity and in frequency, but they are usually not life-threatening. It should be pointed out, too, that much of what appears in the following list may also occur in people who are not infected with the AIDS virus.

• Swollen glands. Lymphadenopathy, characterized by swollen lymph nodes in the neck, armpits, or groin (with or without pain), may occur alone or combined with some of the other symptoms listed below; it is one of the most common signs of infection with the AIDS virus.

• Unexpected and unexplained loss of appetite, and weight loss of more than ten pounds in less than two months.

• Leg weakness, especially difficulty climbing stairs.

• Unexplained fever that has lasted for more than a week.

• Night sweats. Several weeks of waking up drenched with sweat.

• Persistent and unexplained diarrhea. Caused by a protozoan parasite, *Cryptosporidium,* the disorder lasts only a week or two in people with normal immune defenses. In someone infected with the AIDS virus, however, the condition may become chronic, and severe enough to lead to dehydration, malnutrition, and death.

• Persistent, dry coughing, not due to smoking and lasting too long to be attributed to a cold or flu.

• White spots or unusual blemishes in the mouth. Known medically as oral thrush, or candidiasis, this infection of the oral mucous membrane is caused by a yeastlike fungus, *Candida albicans;* it is common and generally benign in infants, but is rare in adults. Two forms occur in adults: one is painless, and is characterized by white patches inside the cheeks, lips, on the gums and soft palate; the other, esophageal candidiasis, is often painful, and the infected person may have difficulty swallowing. Simple candidiasis can be treated by swabbing the mouth with

gentian violet, a dye used to stain cells before examining them under a microscope, or with medicated mouthwashes. The disease can recur, however, and patients must often be treated for life. Its importance to AIDS has been demonstrated in one study of two high-risk groups: in one with oral candidiasis, 86 percent developed AIDS in three months, while none in the other group had the disease after being followed for some twelve months.
• Hairy leukoplakia. A precancerous condition, this is a disease that shows itself with white sores, as well as thickening and overgrowth of the mucous membrane, in the mouth, on the tongue, or in the vagina. It is frequently seen on the tongues of male homosexuals whose immune systems are compromised.
• Shingles. A painful viral disease characterized by blisters that develop along the course of a nerve, shingles is rare in those under fifty who have healthy immune systems. Scientists believe that the virus that causes it lies dormant in the nerve endings, and is suddenly reactivated. Many AIDS patients seem to report an outbreak of shingles before a diagnosis of AIDS is made, and some researchers contend that the skin disorder, when it occurs among male homosexuals, could be a sign of depressed cellular immunity.

In one study, Dr. Alvin Friedman-Kien of New York University Medical Center examined 48 patients — 39 homosexual or bisexual males, 2 female IV-drug users, and 5 men and 2 women who were heterosexual — who had sought medical attention for rashes of shingles on their chests. Blood tests on 35 of the patients revealed antibodies to the AIDS virus, and of the group, 7 developed AIDS within 28 months of the shingles diagnosis; an eighth patient who had originally tested negative tested positive 16 months later, and he developed Kaposi's sarcoma within a month. All 8 were either homosexual or bisexual males between the ages of thirty and forty-eight.[1]
• Lymphoma. A cancer of the lymphatic system, lymphoma can develop before other signs of AIDS are present and, indeed, may be the only clinical manifestation of altered immunity and, thus, the first warning sign of AIDS. In other AIDS patients, however, lymphomas develop along with abnormal growths and infections that are characteristic of AIDS, such as *Pneumocystis carinii* pneumonia.[2]

AIDS

The AIDS stage is the tip of the iceberg. Patients in this last stage are diagnosed as having AIDS if they have a positive blood test for antibodies to the virus, a positive culture for the virus itself, and positive results on lab tests that demonstrate profound immune dysfunction and loss of a specific class of disease-fighting white blood cells called T-4 lymphocytes. They also have one or more of a number of life-threatening opportunistic diseases that are, according to the CDC's current definition of AIDS, "at least moderately indicative of underlying cellular immunodeficiency" that cannot be explained by any cause other than infection with the AIDS virus. The infections and malignancies that accompany AIDS can weaken and disfigure the body and have serious nervous-system consequences ranging from forgetfulness to dementia. It was the appearance of these diseases in otherwise healthy young men that first signaled that a new disease syndrome was taking hold.

• *Pneumocystis carinii* pneumonia. A parasitic infection of the lungs, this disease, before AIDS arrived, was almost exclusively seen in transplant and cancer patients who were receiving immunosuppressive drugs. Also known as pneumocystosis, it is now the most common life-threatening opportunistic infection diagnosed in AIDS patients, with a fatality rate of 25 to 50 percent, despite antimicrobial therapy. Many of those who recover relapse, or eventually die of another opportunistic infection. Its symptoms, similar to any other form of pneumonia, include shortness of breath, dry cough, chills, and fever.

• Cytomegalovirus (CMV) infection. Extremely common among AIDS patients and the general homosexual population, this herpesvirus causes blindness, pneumonia, colitis, and esophagitis. There is no effective treatment for a CMV infection, and while a patient might improve for a time, relapse is quite common.

• Candidiasis in its esophageal form.

• Cryptosporidiosis. Severe diarrhea results from infection with the parasite involved, *Cryptosporidium,* and there is a danger of death.

• Cryptococcosis. Caused by a yeastlike fungus, *Cryptococcus*

neoformans, this disease causes central-nervous-system or other infections. Symptoms include headache, nausea, fever, and blurred vision. Even with treatment, up to 25 percent of patients die.
• Toxoplasmosis. Caused by another protozoan parasite, *Toxoplasma gondii,* this leads to encephalitis (brain inflammation). Symptoms include fever, headache, disordered thinking, lethargy, and seizures. Untreated, the disease is invariably fatal.
• *Mycobacterium avium intracellulare.* Caused by a bacterium related to the one that causes tuberculosis, this disease infects the brain or areas outside the lungs, and is usually fatal. The organism, rarely seen before the discovery of AIDS, has been reported frequently in Haitians with the syndrome. A six-drug treatment is often prescribed, but therapy is generally ineffective since the bacteria strains are especially resistant to antibiotics.
• Herpes simplex viruses. These cause lesions in the mouth and in the rectal and genital areas, or infections in the lungs and gastrointestinal tract. Among individuals with normal immune systems, the lesions are generally mild and temporary, but in AIDS patients, they are more severe, and recur more often.
• Tuberculosis (TB). Not generally regarded as an opportunistic infection, this disease that has plagued humankind since time immemorial now appears with a greater-than-expected frequency in patients with AIDS or those at risk of AIDS, especially IV-drug abusers. Worse, it is far more destructive when it occurs in conjunction with AIDS. Ordinarily, TB is confined to the lungs, but in someone with AIDS, it is apt to spread to the bones, the lymph nodes, the rectum, nerves, and the lining around the heart. Fortunately, TB in AIDS patients responds well to treatment.

The tuberculosis outbreak is, needless to say, a matter of concern, and not only for the AIDS victims. For some years, epidemiologists have been heartened by a slowdown in the number of new TB cases. But the cases arising in AIDS patients may be reversing that trend. Already, some of the areas with the largest number of TB cases (New York City, Florida, California, and Texas) are also the areas with the largest number of AIDS cases. Because TB is so contagious, it may well become the first AIDS-related opportunistic infection to threaten the general public.

• Kaposi's sarcoma. First described in 1872 by a Viennese dermatologist, Moritz Kaposi, this cancer or tumor of the blood- or lymphatic-vessel walls (or both) was, before it started showing up in the very first AIDS patients, rare in the United States; its principal victims had been men over fifty or sixty of Jewish and Italian descent, and organ transplant patients whose immune systems had been suppressed by drugs. (In some equatorial countries of Africa, the incidence of the disease is estimated to be 150 times that of the incidence in the United States; it affects younger patients as well as the elderly there, and tends to be more aggressive than cases seen among the elderly here.)

While it is the most common cancer seen in AIDS patients, for some as-yet-unclear reason Kaposi's sarcoma strikes homosexual men with AIDS far more often than it does other patients with AIDS. (Its incidence in this population, however, is believed to be decreasing, also for unknown reasons.) Rarely life-threatening when it appears in those who develop it in the absence of AIDS, Kaposi's ordinarily is seen as dark blue or purple blotches and bumps that are usually confined to the extremities. But people with AIDS-related Kaposi's are far sicker because the cancer generally spreads to the lymph nodes, the lungs, and the gastrointestinal tract; the disease has also turned up in the brains of some AIDS patients, a rarity before the AIDS outbreak. Although it can kill directly when it results in respiratory failure, the malignancy — which signals an underlying immune deficiency and further debilitates its victims — usually kills indirectly, by opening the way for other opportunistic infections that eventually cause death.

• Dementia and emaciation. The CDC recently added dementia and emaciation to the list of illnesses recognized as confirming a diagnosis of AIDS in patients infected by the AIDS virus. In July 1987, the Social Security Administration, reversing an earlier decision, agreed to use the new, expanded definition of AIDS to determine who qualifies for disability benefits. It is expected that the new classification will increase the number of diagnosed AIDS cases by some 15 percent.

3

What Is the AIDS Virus?

WHEN THE FIRST CASES of Kaposi's sarcoma, *Pneumocystis carinii* pneumonia, and all the other infections began showing up in young, homosexual men in June of 1981, speculation almost immediately focused — as it invariably does when someone comes down with an unexplainable disorder, be it a lethal disease, stomach cramps, or a feeling of malaise — on a virus. There were also some vague allusions to low levels of the male hormone testosterone in the blood of homosexuals, which supposedly, in some mysterious way, made them vulnerable to disease.

There was also much surmising of a less scientific nature — theories based more on morality than on biology, on the wrath of God thundering down on those who refused to accept the dictum, as set forth by a Massachusetts legislator during a debate over a gay rights bill, that God created Adam and Eve, not Adam and Steve. This was not the first time such causality had been alleged: divine fury had also been cited a few years earlier when herpes was cutting a swath through promiscuous heterosexuals. Irrationalism was not confined to straights, either: among some members of the gay community, the equally implausible explanation "the CIA put something in the baths" was commonly expressed. (A similar theme, incidentally, was picked up a few years into the AIDS outbreak, when two Soviet newspapers alleged that the causative agent of AIDS was genetically engineered at the U.S. Army's Fort Detrick, Maryland, laboratories as part of a biological-warfare experiment. American officials, who have characterized the stories as repugnant attempts to sow hatred and suspicion of Americans among the Soviet people, speculate that they began because Fort Detrick, formerly the Army's biological-warfare development center, is now being used for some AIDS-related research.)

The far more reasonable suspicion, a new virus (at least new to the Western world), was soon confirmed when researchers isolated the AIDS virus some two years after the first cases of the disease were diagnosed.

It is true that of the legions of viruses out there — many of which have not yet been identified, and most of which prefer plant, animal, and bacterial targets to humans — countless varieties do not bother humans at all, and, indeed, do us no harm even if they have taken up permanent residence in our bodies. But it is also true that viruses are responsible for more than 60 percent of the sickness that shows up in the developed countries alone (compared to around 15 percent caused by bacteria). The litany of those virally caused ills is a fairly familiar one: flu, measles, mumps, gastroenteritis, rabies, bronchitis, chicken pox, polio, hepatitis, cold sores, genital herpes, smallpox, yellow fever, even some forms of cancer, and perhaps rheumatoid arthritis, multiple sclerosis, and congenital heart disease.

With such a viral track record, why not a virus in AIDS? Why not. Something was obviously attacking a select group of individuals, touching off the sarcomas, the parasite-caused pneumonia, the raging infections caused by germs that in the past had not been responsible for any serious illness, and, beneath it all, the disorder shared by each of those first victims: a failed immune system, the body's first line of defense against disease. But what kind of virus was creating such devastation? And why just homosexuals?

A baffled Centers for Disease Control, aware that it was witnessing the start of a peculiar epidemic the likes of which had never been seen before in the United States, (or anywhere else in the modern world, for that matter), tried to get some answers. The agency assigned a task force of some 30 researchers, led by Dr. James Curran, to analyze whatever 300 other investigators looking into every aspect of the mysterious disease (200 of them in New York City alone) could come up with.

"The scientific interest in this," said Curran at the time, "is enormous."

Among the many early tries was a CDC survey of 300 males, one of the most meticulous case control studies ever attempted. Every detail — medical histories, backgrounds, life-styles — on 50 AIDS patients, all homosexual men, was gathered up. For each of the 50 there were 5 "controls" (healthy men of the same age), 4 of them homosexual and 1 heterosexual, on whom identical data were collected. What the surveyors were looking for was a consistent difference between cases and controls that might offer a clue to the cause of the epidemic.

They managed to turn up two: the men with AIDS had been more sexually active with a large number of different partners, and they had contracted venereal diseases more often. (It is not uncommon for a promiscuous homosexual to have a thousand different partners over a twenty-year span, or fifty partners a year.) The predominance of this group among AIDS cases tended to support the idea that AIDS was also a sexually transmitted disease, undoubtedly caused by some microorganism that gets into the body, probably in infected semen transferred through oral-anal contact, or through anal intercourse, which creates tears in the fragile lining of the rectum. There was precedent for such conjecture: hepatitis B, a known virus-caused disease that attacks the liver and that is also a chronic infector of gay men, is also spread by such an intimate exchange of infected body fluids. Moreover, the researchers suggested, the promiscuous men would probably encounter that organism, whatever it was, repeatedly; as a result, their immune systems would be overwhelmed, leaving them vulnerable to all manner of infections.

Indeed, another study, in Los Angeles, soon afterward buttressed the suspicion that the disease was being transmitted sexually: 9 of the sexual partners of 19 AIDS victims had had sex with other homosexual men who subsequently developed the disease.[1] There were other theories. One was that the recreational drug isobutyl nitrite, known on the street as poppers and widely used among homosexuals as an alleged aphrodisiac, impaired the immune system and thus made it difficult to fight off the opportunistic infections. Another was that a hormonelike compound in human semen suppressed immune function when it entered the bloodstream through abrasions in the rectum during anal intercourse.

Even as laboratory studies aimed at identifying the infecting organism were under way, more cases of AIDS were showing up. But now, along with the homosexual victims, there appeared to be other groups involved: intravenous-drug abusers — among them, heterosexual men and women — and Haitian immigrants. In July of 1982, the disease appeared in still another group of people: three hemophiliacs who had been treated with clotting factors derived from blood to prevent bleeding.

Once again, there was a clue from the spread of the hepatitis virus; along with its ability to enter the body through mucous membranes, the virus also gained easy access via needles that were contaminated by infected blood and were shared among heroin users (a common practice). The connection seemed to have been made that whatever it was that was causing AIDS entered the body in much the same way as the hepatitis virus — through intimate sexual contact, and through infected blood or blood products.

How, next, to explain the Haitian cases? No one had any answers at the time, but speculation was that, despite denials to the contrary, male prostitution, as well as female prostitution, was not uncommon, especially in Carrefour, and, indeed, might well have been responsible for the majority of the Haitian cases. (Unfortunately, epidemiologists often blindly accept what the people they interview tell them.)

With the population at risk for AIDS now apparently defined, researchers began to concentrate on finding the organism responsible. At first, attention was focused on two known viruses, both of which seemed capable of overpowering the immune system, and both of which were members of the notorious herpes family. One was the Epstein-Barr virus, which causes infectious mononucleosis and chronic fatigue, and which may be linked to symptom flare-ups in schizophrenics; it was known to be a factor in the development of nasopharyngeal carcinoma (a cancer of the lining of the nose and throat passages) and Burkitt's lymphoma, an aggressive cancer of white blood cells that afflicts mostly children and is prevalent among young men and boys in equatorial Africa. Lymphomas identical or similar to Burkitt's have recently been turning up with increasing frequency in AIDS patients, and, like the African tumors, some reportedly contain Epstein-Barr-virus DNA. During the early stages of the AIDS outbreak, specialists had noted that many of the diseased patients who had Kaposi's sarcoma had high levels of antibodies to the Epstein-Barr virus, a possible sign of having been infected by it. But the link was puzzling because the herpesviruses have probably been living in human beings for many thousands of years, and the sort of immune damage that was showing up in AIDS victims had not been seen before.

The other suspect was cytomegalovirus (CMV), a virus that infects virtually every one of us at one time or another, usually causing a mild reaction. But in those with weak immune systems, a CMV infection can be quite dangerous, affecting the eyes, the central nervous system, the lungs, the gastrointestinal tract, or the liver. Studies have also shown it to be immunosuppressive in some normal individuals. But aside from its adverse effect on the immune system, there was another important side to CMV: it seemed to be endemic among homosexual males. One study, in fact, revealed evidence of prior cytomegalovirus infection in 94 percent of gay men studied, and another, of 10 homosexual men with Kaposi's sarcoma, found signs of exposure to CMV in all of them; 7 of the 10 also had proteins or genetic material from the virus in tissue samples taken from their tumors.

Because the richest source of the virus in the infected men was semen, scientists speculated that since promiscuous gay men had a very high level of exposure to heavy loads of infected semen — and probably before their immune systems had a chance to recover from a previous CMV infection — they could suffer overwhelming, chronic infection and the immune deficiency characteristic of AIDS. Again, though, CMV had not ever given any sign that it was capable of wrecking a human immune system with the fury associated with AIDS.

These viruses and other early theories were ultimately dismissed. Multiple infections with one pathogen, or with several pathogens? No. Many of the AIDS patients had not had previous multiple infections. Infection with a familiar virus, but one that had chosen a different, and unique, route and modus operandi? Unlikely. Most viruses attack only a particular kind of cell, and seem to have well-defined ways of getting into different hosts.

As scientists ruled out the "old virus, new disease" theory, consensus was building toward an entirely new virus — one that had never been seen before in humans — as the cause of AIDS. It turned out they were on the right track.

Before we can understand what the AIDS virus is, some general background on viruses is absolutely essential, for the AIDS virus differs markedly from most others.

To begin with, all viruses are ultramicroscopic parasites that are smaller than the wavelength of visible light. Despite their tinier-than-bacteria size, they can invade a living cell, reproducing there in isolated safety, and freely wreak as much havoc as bacteria, their far larger, disease-causing cousins. But, when they are taken from their host cells and literally pulled apart and analyzed with the modern tools of molecular biology, viruses, for all their apparent viability, are really no different from what might be found in bottles on the shelves of a chemist's laboratory. They are, simply put, mindless packets of biochemicals that cannot do much without a living cell; they cannot reproduce themselves, nor can they be made to reproduce in nutrient cultures, the watery solutions of chemicals that supply the food an organism like a bacterium requires to multiply. Viruses can be made to reproduce within the cells of an appropriate tissue culture, however; and, once they get inside a live cell, whether it is in a laboratory dish or in someone's body, they take over the cell's metabolic machinery and use it to produce many copies of themselves.

It is tempting to describe viruses simply as primitive packages of infectious chemicals. And compared to bacteria, fungi, rickettsias, protozoa, and all the other microorganisms that invade the body and can cause disease, they are. For whether they are classed as lower or higher forms of life, the nonviruses are alive, and are complex, intricate collections of many kinds of molecules, cells and tiny organs that work closely together to carry out all the processes to sustain life: nutrition, growth, and reproduction.

Not so the viruses. First of all, they are far smaller than the other microorganisms — so tiny they can pass unobserved through the pores of filters generally used to trap even the smallest bacteria. Visible only in the glare and intense magnification of an electron beam, rather than the limited light beam of a conventional microscope, viruses, because they are subcellular, because they are essentially composed of but two substances, and because they lack the mechanism to generate their own energy and reproduce, may be classified as nonliving. They are also not alive, technically speaking, because although they are parasites within a cell, they do not really obtain any nourishment from the cell, as living parasites do; nor, since their innards are mere chemicals, do they need any.

But that characterization as nonliving becomes disputable when we consider that the two "mere" chemicals that make up viruses are, in themselves, most important to life as we know it: a core consisting of nucleic acid, which contains the genetic blueprint for making copies of itself; and around the core, a protective protein wrapper (and around that, perhaps another envelope of fat or carbohydrate).

In some viruses, the nucleic acid stored in the core is DNA (deoxyribonucleic acid), the same genetic material whose precisely arranged molecules make up the genes. Genes, the basic units of inheritance that are found in the cells of all living things, determine whether the cells belong in fish or fowl, man or monkey, germ or geranium. Normally, in a living cell, when a new protein is required for some form or function, the segment of the DNA molecule that codes for those things is switched into another nucleic acid, RNA (ribonucleic acid), which then acts as a messenger, heading outside the cell's nucleus into the cytoplasm, where it oversees the production of new protein. In the virus, the DNA codes for more viruses.

But while all living cells contain both DNA and RNA — a biological imperative if the protein-synthesizing machinery is to work — viruses contain either DNA or RNA in their cores, never both. So, a virus has to compensate. When a DNA virus (the herpes and smallpox viruses are examples) inserts itself into a target cell, it usurps the cell's synthesizing machinery, tricking it into reading, and then replicating, the viral DNA, the blueprint for making more virus, as though it were the cell's own DNA. The cell becomes, thus, a virus factory, spewing out viruses, instead of its own essential substances, before it dies.

Sometimes, too, the infected cell's genetic information is so altered that it makes copies of its now flawed self, and this may result in cancer. There are several other variations on this virus-cell theme, depending on the virus. Some viruses destroy the cell's nucleic acid, thereby ensuring that the virus's own nucleic acid will be in total control of the cell's processes; others simply use their DNA to supplement the cell's synthesizing machinery, perhaps by inserting it, something like a fuel additive, into the cell's nucleic acid.

A more elaborate variation occurs, however, when a cell is infected by a virus with an RNA genome; that is, when its blueprint for making new viruses is imprinted not in DNA, as it is in most viruses and in almost all living things, but in RNA. Such a virus, called a retrovirus, is what the AIDS virus turned out to be. And the twist a retrovirus employs to appropriate a cell's assembly line is to reverse the ordinary flow of genetic information with a gene that codes for a unique enzyme, called reverse transcriptase, whose function is to translate the virus's RNA into DNA. (Enzymes are complicated chemical structures that speed up the thousands of changes that occur in our bodies.) This new viral DNA, now called the provirus, is similar to that of the cell it has chosen to invade, and, because of that similarity, is regarded by the cell as its own genetic material.

Once inside the cell, the provirus is treated as a normal piece of the cell's genetic information, and, most important, is integrated into the DNA in the cell's chromosomes, where it may remain dormant for weeks, months, or years. Or, by taking over the cell's metabolic machinery, it may be transcribed into viral RNA, leading to the production of viral proteins and the formation of new virus particles (virions), which bud out of the cell membrane and are released. Moreover, every time the infected cells divide, copies of the provirus are also produced with each division, each one with the potential of replicating by making further RNA copies that may eventually bud out of the daughter cells. Because of its close relationship with a cell, the retrovirus stays on the scene until the cell dies of the infection or is eliminated by the immune system.

Retroviruses have for some time been linked to virtually all the important plant virus diseases, to Rous sarcoma in chickens (named after the American pathologist Peyton Rous, who, in 1911, demonstrated for the first time that some tumors may have a viral origin), and to leukemia, lymphomas, and immune suppression in cats. But it was not until 1978 that the first human retrovirus was isolated — by one of the scientists now in the forefront of AIDS research, and whose name would eventually be inextricably linked to the AIDS virus: Dr. Robert C. Gallo, head of the laboratory of tumor cell biology at the National Cancer Institute (NCI).

The retrovirus that Gallo found came from the cells of two patients — one a black Caribbean woman living in New York, the other a young black man from Georgia. Laboratory studies determined that the retrovirus, when added to normal cells in a culture dish, zeroed in on the disease-fighting white blood cells known as T-lymphocytes, causing the wild overgrowth that is characteristic of a malignancy; Gallo thus named it HTLV, for "human T-cell leukemia/lymphoma virus."

Subsequently, HTLV was shown to be the cause of an adult form of leukemia unusual in the United States but fairly common in southwestern Japan (90 percent of the leukemia patients studied on the island of Kyushu were found to have the virus); there were also pockets of the disease in the southeastern United States, the Caribbean, southern Italy, and parts of Africa and South America. Soon afterward, Gallo and his team discovered another HTLV virus (it was named HTLV-II) in the blood of a patient with hairy-cell leukemia, a rare blood cancer so named because of the hairlike appearance of the malignant cells. (HTLV-II has not yet been actually linked to any disease, while HTLV, renamed HTLV-I, is strongly associated with the adult form of leukemia. Because of the association, however, both retroviruses are classified in a subfamily called oncoviruses, the term used for viruses that cause tumors.)

In 1982, when reports of AIDS cases began pouring into the

CDC, Gallo and Max Essex, a cancer biologist at the Harvard School of Public Health, started speculating that not only was AIDS being caused by a retrovirus, but the retrovirus belonged, perhaps, to this same HTLV family. Gallo, in fact, proposed such a link in February of that year at a conference on AIDS at Cold Spring Harbor, in New York. His reasoning had a sound basis, for the evidence was tantalizing, to say the least. First of all, Essex had found that some retroviruses had been tied not only to leukemia and opportunistic infections in cats, but to an AIDS-like immune suppression. (In October 1986, researchers at the Children's Hospital in Boston reported that a retrovirus was also the possible cause of the mysterious childhood illness Kawasaki disease — the leading cause of acquired heart disease in children and an illness characterized by a unique set of changes in the immune cells of its young victims.) Essex also, in collaboration with Japanese scientists, had found that some people infected with HTLV-I were prone to high rates of opportunistic infections, just as the AIDS victims were.

Moreover, there was the fact that HTLV-I was endemic in two places where AIDS was showing up in big numbers: Haiti and Africa. There was the rare Kaposi's sarcoma in AIDS patients, which, since it affected the skin's blood vessels, might be caused by a virus that attacked the blood cells. (Subsequent investigation ruled this link out, since Kaposi's is not caused directly by the AIDS virus, but results from the immune deficiency, just as the Kaposi's tumors occur in organ transplant patients who receive immunosuppressive drugs to stop their bodies from fighting off the grafts.)

In addition, there were the intriguing similarities in the way AIDS and HTLV-I infection seemed to be transmitted — through sexual intercourse, blood transfusions, and the contaminated needles of drug abusers. Also — like AIDS, it turned out — infection with the HTLV-I virus did not necessarily mean a person would get the disease: it is estimated the virus can hang on in its host in latent form for some forty years, causing the leukemia in only 1 out of 100 persons. (Further epidemiological data also came up with a figure for the number of Japanese carriers of HTLV-I that did not differ very much from the estimated number of AIDS carriers: one million.)

But something else was most important to the oncovirus theory: both of Gallo's retroviruses attacked the so-called T-4 cells — an important group of T-lymphocytes that serve as master controls for the body's immune system — just as the suspected AIDS virus seemed to be doing. (AIDS patients, we now know, have fewer T-4 cells than healthy people.) The difference, it turned out later, was that HTLV-I causes T-cells to proliferate uncontrollably, while the AIDS virus does just the opposite, wrecking the T-cells.

Converting conjecture into fact, however, was not easy. It meant finding the virus in the blood cells of AIDS patients, growing it, preventing it from killing off the culture cells before it could be studied in detail, and then actually proving that it caused disease. The infinitesimal scale on which all of this would have to be done was, quite naturally, somewhat of a drawback. Scientists have to use a measurement known as a millimicron, which amounts to 1 one-millionth of a millimeter, to map their way around viruses and help to identify them. One of the tiniest viruses, for example, is the polio virus; it logs in with a diameter of 10 millimicrons. By contrast, the width of a staphylococcus bacterium is 1,000 millimicrons. Moreover, if viruses were but simple, elongated structures, it would be difficult enough to determine their size; but they come in some convoluted, as well as perfectly geometric, shapes: rods, helixes, filaments, and spheroids that are, on closer scrutiny, really polyhedrons.

The electron microscope, of course, has been invaluable in tracking down viruses (although to the untrained eye some viruses, when viewed under the enormous magnification of the instrument, are but uninteresting, grainy smudges). And it was unlikely, given the suspect's apparent similarities to other known viruses, that it would be an agent too small to see and photograph. Finding it, since researchers were quite sure it was there somewhere, was a matter of time: something that was bound to happen after enough blood and serum samples from AIDS patients were painstakingly cleansed of contaminants and various other cellular chemicals, then scrutinized for antibodies to the virus and for evidence of reverse-transcriptase activity.

Gallo's initial efforts to establish a link between AIDS and HTLV were promising, but not definitive. Apparently, there was some evidence of the presence of a retrovirus — in the form of reverse-transcriptase activity — when he mixed cells from AIDS patients with fresh T-cells; but further probing for either HTLV-I or HTLV-II turned up nothing in the way of a virus. The limited action Gallo had been getting, however, seemed to indicate that something was leaving a footprint in his samples — something that looked like HTLV-I or HTLV-II, but was not either. Essex had also detected antibodies to HTLV-I in a high percentage of AIDS patients (but not in healthy, matched control subjects); and, later, Gallo turned up HTLV-I genes in the DNA of T-cells from two AIDS patients. He also isolated the virus itself in one patient.

In May 1983, the two scientists published the results of their HTLV-AIDS research in the journal *Science*. But right alongside was a report by a team from the Institut Pasteur in Paris that seemed to nail down the true culprit. The French researchers told how they had separated a virus they had not ever seen before from a swollen lymph node of a thirty-three-year-old homosexual patient suffering from lymphadenopathy syndrome, a disorder that is regarded as an early symptom of ARC. They named it LAV, for "lymphadenopathy-associated virus."

It is interesting to note that the new virus — which was similar to, but also distinct from, HTLV — received scant attention at the time. (Gallo, incidentally, was the so-called referee — the scientist who reviews articles for a journal and gives the go-ahead for publication.) There was, moreover, a good deal of skepticism. For one thing, the electron microscope photographs were of such relatively poor quality that technicians thought the French scientists had been mistaken in characterizing their virus as a retrovirus. Another problem was that the French had isolated only a single virus, and so it was unclear whether it was a cause of AIDS or of one of the accompanying infections.

Still, the Pasteur team pressed its case, at the first European AIDS conference in Naples in June, and later at an HTLV conference at Cold Spring Harbor, New York. Dr. Luc Montagnier of the French team recalled that the reception he got from American researchers at Cold Spring Harbor was not especially cordial. Gallo was one of those who seemed skeptical. "He asked me if it were really a retrovirus," said Montagnier.

"After the meeting was over, he told me, 'I don't know if you're right or wrong, but I'm going to work on it for six months, and if it turns out you're right, then I'll tell everyone.'"[2]

But Gallo, understandably, was more concerned with his own work than with the French discovery. For one thing, gay activists had been criticizing the Reagan administration for not moving fast enough against AIDS. As a result, there was now about $12 million in public money behind the National Cancer Institute effort to combat AIDS (compared to $425,000 in France). And there was Gallo himself, forty-seven years old, as feisty and flamboyant as Luc Montagnier was quiet and reserved, an NCI superstar who for more than a decade had pushed his lab to one brilliant achievement after another in cell biology, molecular biology, and virology. A furiously driven competitor ("I want to be something better than the best I've ever seen"), he had a predilection for bravura that sometimes paid off: when he became the NCI's top AIDS researcher in 1982, he vowed that the cause of the disease would be found in two years.

Gallo had also tested the French virus, but his first efforts to get any reverse-transcriptase activity with it were apparently fruitless. Working with a second sample, which was sent to Gallo in September of 1983, the NCI lab detected some reverse-transcriptase activity — a sign that the virus in the samples was a retrovirus — when they added the virus to fresh cells. But in a few days, the cells deteriorated, and virus production quit. Apparently, the virus was destroying the culture cells faster than the researchers could analyze them, a situation somewhat akin to plowing under a garden that has just begun to bloom. Gallo said he put the cultures in the freezer.

A few months later, Gallo's team had the nettling culture problem solved. While the French were still getting their samples by standard, time-consuming culture methods, Mikulas Popovic, a cell biologist in the NCI lab, was developing a new line of cells, which he called the H9 line, that could be easily infected with the suspected new virus. But more important, the cell line could be infected without being destroyed. The breakthrough was the key to growing large quantities of virus for study, and to the subsequent development of a test that could screen for antibodies to the virus in the blood of AIDS victims.

In May 1984, Gallo and his collaborators published four papers in the journal *Science* reporting that they had indeed isolated the new virus in samples from 48 patients with AIDS. Moreover, antibodies to the virus were found in 90 percent of all AIDS patients tested, and in 80 percent of those with symptoms that often precede the disease. By contrast, less than one-half of 1 percent of the apparently healthy homosexuals tested as controls had the antibodies.

The virus that Gallo and his team found was remarkably similar to LAV, which itself was, again, similar to, but clearly distinct from, the earlier HTLV specimens. Because it shared morphological, biological, and immunological characteristics with other earlier members of the HTLV family, Gallo and his colleagues called the virus HTLV-III, making a slight change in the original meaning of HTLV: instead of "human T-cell leukemia/lymphoma virus," the letters now stood for "human T-cell lymphotropic virus," referring to the predilection all the HTLV viruses have for T-cells. Three months later, at the University of California at San Francisco, Jay Levy and his collaborators isolated an AIDS virus from AIDS patients. They called theirs ARV, for AIDS-related virus.

Because the new virus was not turning up in blood samples from healthy heterosexuals (less than 1 percent, for instance, showed any evidence of HTLV-III infection), and because antibodies to the virus were indeed showing up in the blood of most AIDS patients and homosexual males with symptoms of early AIDS infection, researchers were now certain they had found their culprit.

In fact, on April 23, shortly before the Gallo team's AIDS papers were published in *Science*, Gallo and Margaret Heckler, secretary of the Department of Health and Human Services, appeared at a news conference to announce what Heckler prematurely called "the triumph of science over a dread disease."

The Pasteur team was miffed, and not without justification. For one thing, the day before Heckler's optimistic pronouncement, the *New York Times* ran a front-page story in which James O. Mason, head of the CDC (which had been collaborating with the French scientists) noted that newly acquired data indicated strongly that the virus isolated at Pasteur in 1983 was the cause of AIDS. For another, about two weeks before the news conference, the British journal *Lancet* had carried another report from the French stating that they had found more LAV viruses in AIDS patients; it, too, had gone largely unnoticed by the American press. Even some of Gallo's own colleagues criticized him for his apparent attempt to preempt the French and his reluctance to share his results with other U.S. scientists before publication.

But that was what the story of the virus hunt had been. Not only was it a tale of false leads and bitter disappointments, blind luck and gut instinct, drudgery and inspiration, but it was also one that was often being played out in an environment of unfriendly competition, arrogance, scientific elitism, and strong egos. (According to a report in *Science* in November 1985, to Gallo and his associates, Mason's announcement looked like a deliberate attempt by the CDC and the Pasteur scientists to steal his thunder. "Relations between Gallo and the CDC were already strained," the journal noted, "and Gallo was competing with the French researchers to nail down the cause of AIDS." Insofar as Mason was concerned, he said he had not seen Gallo's papers when he was interviewed by the *Times*, and Pasteur officials denied any part in Mason's announcement.)[3]

There comes a genuine break in the story at this point: a series of unfortunate disputes of the sort that invariably result when highly competitive human beings, in this instance, scientists, are going for the gold. In the case of AIDS, the gold was (1) credit for discovering the virus, (2) patent rights in any AIDS test and a share of the royalties when and if the test was developed and marketed, and (3) perhaps a Nobel Prize. The disputes spawned more tension, mistrust, charges, and countercharges among researchers than ordinarily occur (and in the sometimes grant-and-glory-hungry world of research, that's no mean achievement); and for a time, they seemed to put a crimp in the pace of AIDS research.

One difficulty was what to call the virus, now that three research teams had isolated, and named, their own. The various isolates that were being extracted from AIDS and ARC patients appeared to be quite similar to one another, and if indeed they were, it seemed logical to select one name to cover them all.

But it is not as simple as all that. To molecular biologists, similarity is determined by the way the viruses' nucleotides — the chemical building blocks, or subunits, that make up the viruses' genetic blueprint — are arranged. In the case of the AIDS isolates, analysis generally confirmed that although there seemed to be little doubt that all were very closely related, there were sometimes subtle, but important, variations in their genetic makeups (which, as we will see later, present difficulties for the development of a vaccine against AIDS). Gallo has pointed out, for example, that the genetic sequences of his virus and the French virus differed by about 1.5 percent; 6 percent of the ARV building blocks were found to be different when that virus was compared to HTLV-III. Earlier, he had bristled when I asked him whether he had compared HTLV-III to LAV thoroughly.

While the formal name of the AIDS virus, no matter what it was, would mean little to patients or to the doctors treating them, it was still important from a scientific standpoint, because a name could place the virus squarely into a specific family. And the family that Gallo had placed it in was the HTLV one he had discovered.

The French, it turned out, were not especially thrilled at that. "Gallo was the father of HTLV-I and HTLV-II," said Luc Montagnier. "So, it's natural that he should want the new virus to be a continuation of the same family."

In an attempt to resolve the dispute over the virus's name, members of the human retrovirus subcommittee of the International Committee on Taxonomy of Viruses proposed in May of 1986 that it be called HIV, for "human immunodeficiency virus." This followed the rules of retrovirus nomenclature, which begin with the host's species (*human*), denote a characteristic of the virus (*immunodeficiency*), and end with *virus*. According to Jay Levy, a member of the subcommittee, the group avoided AIDS in the name because several doctors had written to suggest that the term was too frightening to the public. Also, the virus attacks brain and other cells besides T-cells in the body, and avoiding the allusion to the T-cells in the name of Gallo's virus took note of that.[4] Calling the virus HIV also skirted the issue of who the discoverer was.

There seemed, however, to be no chance that the new name would catch on. Gallo and Harvard's Max Essex both announced they had no intention of adopting HIV. (Levy and Montagnier both agreed to endorse the subcommittee's proposed change.) Gallo pointed out that a computer search had shown that 95 percent of scientific publications called the virus HTLV-III and that only a handful of the subcommittee members actually worked with the AIDS virus. Said Gallo: "Those of us working in the field are the ones to decide what to call the virus. I don't think [HIV is] a particularly good name. A lot of viruses cause immune deficiency — cytomegalovirus, Epstein-Barr. I will never refer to Dr. Montagnier's virus as HIV-I."[5] (At an international AIDS symposium in Paris in June of 1986, Montagnier opened a presentation with words that still left the matter somewhat murky: "Three and a half years after its discovery, the AIDS retrovirus — LAV, HTLV-III, ARV, HIV — has revealed most of its characteristics.")

The controversy over the name was overshadowed, however, by an incident that further heated the bitter rivalry between the American and French AIDS scientists. In 1985, the Pasteur team sued the National Institutes of Health and the U.S. government, charging Gallo's team with breach of contract for using samples of virus and research data supplied by Pasteur, both as a standard while they were working on isolating the HTLV-III virus and to develop the AIDS antibody-detection kit that is currently being used by blood banks and hospitals to screen blood for evidence of AIDS infection. Gallo had agreed to use the materials for research only, and though his group took out a patent on the blood test (on behalf of the federal government), he vehemently denied using the French virus samples when the NCI group developed its test, adding that he had access to many samples of his own virus. The French, he said, were exaggerating their role. "We helped them a lot more than they helped us," Gallo told a reporter.[6]

That probably was not only bombast. Many scientists believe — and not without justification — that although both teams have made enormous contributions, it was the sweeping range and elegance of Gallo's research that resulted in far more detailed information about the virus and that provided, even though his team was beaten into print by the French, the overwhelming evidence that the new virus caused AIDS. Gallo has insisted, moreover, that the French were able to grow and identify their virus only after he sent them the essential biological tools — notably T-cell growth factor, an earlier Gallo discovery that made it possible to study human T-cells in tissue culture for prolonged periods and that has helped bring about many advances in immunology. Without Gallo's persistence, it appears, the French viruses may well have remained, as one researcher put it, scientific curiosities.

The Pasteur scientists had a point, though, arguing that they, and not Gallo, had actually discovered the AIDS virus. And they insisted on recognition of that fact, demanding not only a share of the royalties the United States collected from sales of the blood tests by licensees, but also permission for the French to license firms to sell the test without any legal hassles from the United States. (The U.S. Patent and Trademark Office had apparently ignored Pasteur's request in December 1983 for a patent on an AIDS antibody test, a denial Gallo said was based on the fact that the French had not come up with a working blood test.)

Apart from the scientific recognition, the royalties would be uplifting: 5 percent a year on $40 million in sales of the tests. (It should be noted that Gallo receives no royalties from the patent; the money is paid to the U.S. Treasury.) Gallo's feeling was that it was immaterial who actually discovered the AIDS virus, and that his lab's achievement in growing it in large quantities first was the crucial step toward developing a workable blood test. As Donald Macdonald, acting assistant secretary of health, put it, "We had the science first." Charles Lipsey, a patent lawyer for Pasteur, disagreed. "What matters is who made the invention first," he said.[7]

The situation worsened with the revelation — actually an admission by Gallo and his colleagues — that they had mistakenly published electron micrographs of the French virus in one of the key papers that reported the discovery of the American virus. The embarrassing admission came in a legend correction in the journal *Science* (18 April 1986) in which Gallo and members of his team acknowledged that a panel of photographs labeled HTLV-III "was inadvertently composed" from photographs of a culture that had been "transiently" infected with a sample of LAV provided by Montagnier's lab. Lawyers for the Pasteur scientists seized on the gaffe, charging that the fact that electron micrographs were taken of the French virus added to the circumstantial evidence that Gallo's team obtained vital information from the Pasteur materials and, contrary to what the U.S. government had been saying, had been doing work on LAV. If Gallo had his own virus, the French argued, why, then, was he growing and photographing LAV, the original samples of which, he had claimed, were too small and too difficult to grow?

Gallo's response was typical of a man short of fuse: "What were we supposed to do with the virus, eat it?"[8] Photographing the virus was standard lab procedure, he said, and the only agreement was not to use it for commercial purposes. Furthermore, Gallo maintained, he could prove conclusively that his team had other electron micrographs of the HTLV-III virus — as well as evidence of reverse-transcriptase activity — dating back as far as February of 1983, more than six months before the LAV samples arrived from Pasteur.

This "Tempest in a Test Tube," as the *Wall Street Journal* headlined the story, was partially resolved when a federal claims court judge dismissed Pasteur's plea for recognition as the discoverer of the AIDS virus on the grounds that the court had no jurisdiction over the research agreement between Pasteur and NCI. The decision left the patent dispute still unresolved, although in June 1986, the U.S. Patent and Trademark Office acknowledged that the Pasteur group indeed had a rival claim to the antibody-test patent and were entitled to a formal hearing.

The rift ended in March 1987 when President Ronald Reagan and Prime Minister Jacques Chirac of France announced that researchers from their countries had agreed to share both credit for the discovery of the AIDS virus and patent rights to the blood test; moreover, they agreed to refer to the virus as HIV, and to donate most of the royalties from the test to a new foundation for AIDS research and education.

(Gallo and Montagnier had earlier shared something else related to their virus research: both men won 1986 Albert Lasker Awards for medical research and public service — significant honors if only for the fact that forty-two previous winners have gone on to win Nobel Prizes. Gallo picked up his Lasker, his second, for finding the AIDS retrovirus in the blood of AIDS patients, and for his work in getting it to grow; Montagnier was honored for discovering the retrovirus.)

By now the AIDS virus had been isolated and grown in human cell cultures, and it was being detected, either directly or through antibody action against it, in the blood of AIDS patients but not in that of healthy heterosexuals. Much more had yet to be learned about its natural history, however. Was it, for example, linked to any existing family of viruses?

Further detailed analyses of the virus's insides began to make it evident that although the AIDS virus is a member of the HTLV family, it is not a human leukemia virus, as was first thought. Its connection to cancer — the Kaposi's sarcoma in AIDS patients, for instance — is, as we noted earlier, an indirect one; that is, it is a cause of the immune deficiency that causes the tumor that often accompanies AIDS. Suffice it to say that it has several features in common with the other HTLV members — a generalization that is truly for the best when the lay reader considers what Gallo's team originally gave as one arcane example of that commonality: "a reverse transcriptase with a high molecular weight (100,000) and a preference for $Mg2+$ as the divalent cation for optimal enzymatic activity."[9]

The AIDS virus was soon being more accurately described as a member of the retrovirus subfamily of lentiviruses, not the retrovirus subfamily of oncoviruses. Lentiviruses (whose DNA sequences resemble those in the AIDS virus) do not cause cancer, but of the three that are known, one is responsible for brain infections in sheep, another for infectious anemia in horses, and the third for encephalitis in goats. Until the AIDS connection, none of the lentiviruses — also called slow viruses, because several years may pass between the time they infect a host and the appearance of symptoms — was thought to cause human disease. For that reason, and because they could not be readily transmitted to small lab animals for study, little was known about them. (One of the human diseases known to be caused by a slow virus is kuru, a fatal nervous system disease seen almost exclusively among a single tribe in New Guinea, and spread by rites associated with cannibalism.) This much, however, was certain: when lentiviruses infect domestic animals, they become so lethal and unresponsive to drugs that the animals have to be slaughtered.

The similarities between what the known lentiviruses did in animals and what the AIDS virus did in humans were striking. The AIDS virus, like the other lentiviruses, quite often takes a while to show itself (that is, by displaying symptoms of the debilitating disease). Both the AIDS virus and other lentiviruses produce neurological impairment since both can infect brain cells. Both also infect T-cells, although which of those cells the lentiviruses prefer, and how much effect they exert on the cells, differ from species to species. Two of the lentiviruses, the caprine arthritis encephalitis virus (which attacks goats) and the visna virus (the sheep virus), apparently home in on two types of large white blood cells: monocytes and macrophages, both of which ingest cell debris and bacteria. Besides infecting T-cells, the AIDS virus also attacks monocytes and macrophages.

Still another parallel may be drawn from the visna virus. Its name is apropos when discussing the enfeebling effects of AIDS: *visna* is Icelandic for "wasting," and *visna* is what the sheep disease was called when it suddenly appeared in Iceland in the 1930s, killing some 150,000 animals by 1952. Centuries of isolation, it was speculated, made the sheep particularly susceptible to the virus. The animals were, thus, easy targets, and their situation could be likened to the relative isolation and vulnerability of the homosexual and IV-drug-abusing communities that were first hit by the human AIDS virus. Some of the sheep disease's symptoms even mimic those of AIDS: brain inflammation, the infected lymph nodes of lymphadenopathy, and susceptibility to infections, the most common of which is an acute pneumonia caused by a bacterium that probably lived in Icelandic sheep before visna virus came along.[10]

4

Where Did the Virus Originate?

WHEN THE FIRST HALF-DOZEN U.S. cases of AIDS were reported in Los Angeles in 1981, scientists at the Centers for Disease Control were convinced they were looking at a new disease because they had never seen anything destroy an immune system so fast. But as the epidemic grew, they started changing their minds. It now appeared that AIDS was new only to the Western world, that it had originated in central Africa, and that the virus that caused it was perhaps an evolutionary descendant of one that had existed in monkeys for as long as 50,000 years, one that had mutated enough to enable it to jump species fairly recently and infect human cells. There was also the possibility that the virus had existed in humans in central Africa for hundreds of thousands of years, causing only minor symptoms in isolated groups until it spread more widely later on as infected people began migrating to the cities and came into contact with previously unexposed and vulnerable populations.

Whatever the scenario, evidence began to accumulate that the AIDS virus, or some variation of it, was, in fact, present in Africa at least a decade or two before the first U.S. cases were detected. One retrospective clue came during the 1970s when various AIDS-like symptoms were observed in some western-Africans who came to Europe. Another sign of something amiss came when researchers began noticing that the incidence and severity of Kaposi's sarcoma in central Africa was changing. Back in the seventies, the skin cancer that is now associated with AIDS accounted for up to 20 percent of all cancers in Africa and was quite rare in the rest of the world. But though prevalent in Africa, it was relatively mild. For instance, of 600 African Kaposi's patients studied at the time by Alexander Templeton, a pathologist at Rush–Presbyterian–St. Luke's Medical Center in Chicago, fewer than 5 percent were afflicted with the most aggressive form of the disease, one that kills in a matter of months. Most of the victims suffered from a type that was sometimes disfiguring, but rarely life-threatening. But that changed. The prevalent Kaposi's sarcoma in Africa these days is usually fatal, and its incidence has reportedly quadrupled in some areas over the past fifteen years. Templeton speculated not long ago that the rapid spread of the deadlier form of Kaposi's sarcoma was proof that an AIDS virus, with its coincidental link to Kaposi's, mutated sometime after 1972 into a more savage form. It might have been only a small shift in the original virus's makeup, but it apparently was enough to transform an obscure and rarely lethal disease into something virulent and widespread.

The first real evidence of the virus's new savagery came in March of 1985, in a report in *Science* by Robert Gallo and an international team of collaborators. Studying frozen blood samples taken from 42,000 Ugandans between August 1972 and July 1973, Gallo analyzed 75 at random and found that nearly 65 percent of the children and 48 percent of the adults carried antibodies to the HTLV-III virus, which meant they had all been exposed to it. Since there had been no outbreak of anything resembling AIDS in the years before the samples were taken, Gallo and others theorized that the virus must have mutated in the mid- to late 1970s, roughly when it began to break out of Africa.

Another reason AIDS may not have erupted into an epidemic until it came to the United States in the late seventies, Gallo suggested, was that Ugandans could have been infected with a virus just as potent as the current version, but for some reason were genetically resistant to it and thus able to harbor it without showing signs of serious disease. Other studies found some evidence of the virus — that is, antibodies to it or something closely related to it — in blood samples taken even earlier: in 2 of 544 samples collected in Upper Volta in 1963, and in another sample drawn in Léopoldville in 1959. Although the total number of positives in all the samples was relatively small, it was, nevertheless, a strong sign that the AIDS virus had gained a foothold.

Many researchers believe that HTLV-I and HTLV-III were the products of a mutation, and that the original source was an African monkey. That an animal should be blamed for starting such a disease should come as no surprise. In his famous 1911 monograph on the hookworm, parasitologist Arthur Looss addressed the issue in this way:

> We often do not know the special behavior and special development of a certain intestinal worm of Man, but if the study of related forms living in animals were undertaken we should attain a fair certainty as to what the truth will be. The familiarity with the parasites of animals enables the observer, in many cases, to say at once whether a theory set up with regard to a parasite of Man is intrinsically probable, i.e., whether or not it can be correct. What I wish here to emphasize is that a correct knowledge of the diseases of man caused by worms, and all that is connected with them, is the more difficult to attain the more the parasites of animals are ignored.[1]

While scientists will probably never pinpoint the identity of the AIDS virus's immediate progenitor, they do know that the disease is endemic in the central African nations of Zaire, Burundi, Uganda, Rwanda, Tanzania, and Kenya, and that a species of monkey plentiful in the area, the African green, carries a virus called STLV-III (for simian T-lymphotropic virus) that has been shown to be remarkably similar to HTLV-III both in structure and in the blood cells it prefers. The greens, which also pass along a hemorrhagic disease called Ebola Valley fever to humans, do not get sick from STLV-III as other primates do, probably because they have some protective mechanism. Thus, they could have been carrying the virus long before it began infecting humans. The green monkeys also seem to have a partiality to another facet of AIDS: besides STLV-III, they carry an earlier version, STLV-I, which is, as might be suspected, another look-alike of HTLV-I, the original member of Gallo's virus family.

Scientists at the New England Primate Center in Southborough, Massachusetts, discovered the simian virus when rhesus monkeys — a common research species whose immune systems are very similar to those of humans — began dying in their cages of a mysterious disease with symptoms much like those of AIDS. While the scientists did not know how the virus got into the monkey colony, they speculated on how it was spread: through homosexual and heterosexual relations, as well as the spraying of urine, common occurrences when the monkeys were caged. (The incidence of the disease dropped once the animals were housed separately.) Signs of the virus had first been detected in the monkeys' tissues, but although scientists suspected that some kind of virus was causing the disease, they were unable to isolate it and prove its causative connection.

That came in September of 1984, when the Southborough researchers cultured the HTLV-III look-alike from a monkey with the AIDS-like syndrome and injected it into six healthy monkeys. Within two weeks of inoculation, the virus was isolated from the monkeys' blood. Within 120 to 160 days, four of the animals became deathly ill from immunologic abnormalities, wasting, weight loss, and diarrhea. One of the two remaining monkeys developed a pre-AIDS-like syndrome of wasting and swollen lymph glands 200 days after inoculation, while the other remained clinically well. Lab tests and subsequent autopsy reports clinched the connection to AIDS: the four immunodeficient monkeys had drastic losses in the number of T-cells, losses that persisted until shortly before the animals died; the ability of the lymphocytes to fight infection also dropped markedly, and three of the monkeys died of disease caused by adenovirus, a DNA-containing virus that causes respiratory tract infections, and that has been implicated in the formation of tumors and opportunistic infections common to AIDS. The four monkeys also suffered serious central-nervous-system damage — all of them had primary retroviral encephalitis — and STLV-III was isolated from the brain tissue of two, a significant finding because of the presence of HTLV-III in the brains of

AIDS patients and the mounting evidence that the AIDS virus attacks the nervous system more often and with more ferocity than previously believed.

There were some differences, however, between the human and monkey diseases. For one thing, the monkeys' lymph nodes were not enlarged, as they are in human patients. Another difference was in the development period of the two diseases: the monkey disorder had an incubation period of only a few weeks, while the incubation of AIDS in humans can take months or years. One explanation for this, according to Dr. Norman Letvin of the primate center, was that the young, immature immune systems of the monkeys may have been especially vulnerable to the virus; also, massive doses were given, which may have speeded up the onset of the disease.

Despite the differences, the overall results of the research provided an animal model for human AIDS, paving the way for a viable way to study AIDS treatments and potential vaccines in lab animals. "This helps us look at AIDS in a different perspective," Letvin commented after the initial test. "AIDS is no longer a unique disease in man with no parallels in the animal world. The fact is, there are other diseases in nature that have striking similarities to AIDS."[2] The monkey model was especially good news because the other animal models that have been used, such as feline leukemia, are only distantly related to AIDS, while the link that had been established between the STLV-III disease and human AIDS was indisputable. The fact that the disease occurred in the rhesus monkeys was also providential. Researchers have logged an enormous number of experiments with the animals, and they are far more accessible than many other primates, such as chimpanzees, which are an endangered species and virtually unavailable for research.

5

How Does the Virus Cause Infection?

IDENTIFYING THE ORIGIN of the AIDS virus and which group of retroviruses it belonged to was, of course, important if scientists were to determine how it caused disease. But more work lay ahead before a fuller understanding of the infective process could be gained, and there were a multitude of questions still to be answered: Exactly how did the AIDS virus touch off the rapid-fire multiplication of itself that was its hallmark? How, precisely, did it go about killing cells? Why, sometimes, did it not cause any ill effects in its victims for years? Where in the body did it hide when it was not hosted by, and immobilizing, the T-cells? What other cells was it able to infect? How did the virus gain access to the brain in so many cases? Did it interact with other viruses, or with other cofactors, to make infection easier, or to worsen the disease? What drove this virus, what made it tick?

We have seen that the AIDS virus is a retrovirus, one that stores its genetic program in the nucleic acid RNA instead of DNA and that uses a special enzyme, reverse transcriptase, to make a DNA copy of its RNA program. The conversion enables the retrovirus to insinuate itself easily into DNA-formatted cells, turning them into factories for more viruses. But before any virus can enter and infect a healthy cell, its specially tailored protein coat has to match receptors on the cell in a sort of lock-and-key arrangement; the key is a protein protuberance on the virus's outer membrane, and the lock is a receptor site on the cell's surface. When the fit is perfect, the virus can inject its genetic material into the cell and infect it. When it is not, the variations in the configuration of either the viral key or the cellular lock prevent the virus from gaining entry. This precise meshing explains why viruses are so choosy about which species and which cell type within that species they will infect.

Some viruses, like the hepatitis A virus (also called infectious hepatitis, and not as severe as hepatitis B), enter the body through contaminated food and water, then fit receptors on the epithelial cells lining the digestive tract. Flu viruses can be transmitted through food or by kissing because they, too, can lock on to epithelial cells.

The AIDS virus ties primarily on to T-4 cells — a linkup that, incidentally, contributes to the virus's relatively low level of contagiousness: since the T-4 cells are not usually found in the digestive tract, transmission of the AIDS virus through contaminated foods is highly unlikely. But T-4 cells are in plentiful supply in the human immune system, representing more than 60 percent of the body's lymphocytes in well individuals. And it is amid such abundance that the AIDS virus is able to proliferate almost effortlessly.

The human immune system, where the AIDS virus begins most of its damage, is an incredibly complex biological network of organs, fluids, and cells that guards against disease. No one of the body's principal organs, however, actually controls the immune system. It is, in a sense, a biological collective — a cooperative unit of highly specialized individual members, each with its own job assignment, and each in constant communication with the others, through an intricate, chemical signal system. For our purpose, which is to understand how the AIDS virus disrupts this biochemical society, it is probably enough to say that its major components are three groups of white blood cells (about 1 trillion out of the total 100 trillion cells that circulate through the body), all of which originate in the bone marrow.

The phagocytes — which include "scavenger" cells, the macrophages — are in one group. When the immune system is functioning properly, these large cells engulf and break down viruses, bacteria, and cellular debris in a process known as phagocytosis.

The T-lymphocytes and the B-lymphocytes comprise the remaining two groups of white cells; between them, they represent the immune system's major resistance to the wide range of bacteria and viruses that enter the body and may cause disease. Each type of lymphocyte is stored in the major organs of the lymphatic system — the lymph nodes and the spleen — and when needed, circulates through the blood and the lymph, the colorless, watery fluid of dissolved salts and proteins that bathes the tissues.

The B-cells, by dividing and redividing many times over the course of several days, produce thousands of different specific antibodies, the Y-shaped protein molecules that stream to the site of an infection and either mark an invading organism for destruction by other cells or neutralize or destroy the invader themselves. Each B-cell has the ability to make just one kind of antibody, and each antibody is engineered to bind onto just one kind of intruding bacterium or virus. Because each intruder has its own identifying chemical substances, antigens, on its surface, when one of these intruders gets into the body, only the antibodies that precisely match the antigenic site attach to it, ball-and-socket fashion, thus marking it as a target. Once the intruder is destroyed and the immune response returns to normal, some of the B-cells hold on to a "memory" of the antigen in the event it should reappear; if it does, more antibodies are made against that particular antigen. What is even more remarkable about B-cells is that there are enough different types to produce specific antibodies against just about anything that gets into the body.

The T-cells play more of a leadership role than the B-cells. They mature in the thymus, a tiny gland that is nestled beneath the breastbone, and come in several forms. Each has a different function, but together, they really control the immune response. One kind is the cytotoxic T-cell (also called a killer T-cell), which directly destroys the antigens or the infected cells that have been invaded by a virus. Another is the suppressor T-cell; this one moderates or turns off the immune response by slowing up the B-cells and the killer T-cells, effectively putting a stop to the body's counterattack when the infection abates.

Another type of T-cell is the helper-T, the so-called T-4 cell, which is the one the AIDS virus preferentially attacks. (The numeral 4 associated with this cell identifies a protein molecule on the cell's surface.) Its job is to correctly identify an antigen, stimulate the B-cells to make antibodies, and activate the killer T-cells. The T-4 cell accomplishes that chore by secreting hormonelike substances called lymphokines, which serve as a messenger between it, the B-cells, and the killer T-cells. Stimulated by lymphokines, the B-cells divide and secrete antibodies, and the killer cells go into action. The T-4 cell is, thus, the most vital member of the immune team, for its mission is both to survey the body for signs of danger and to get an immune response under way when warranted.

Because of such superb teamwork, it is easy to understand why language ordinarily applied to human traits and endeavors comes easily when talking about the immune system. (It is hard not to anthropomorphize viruses when describing their behavior. One newspaper science reporter recently characterized the AIDS virus as "diabolical" and "selfish," while another described viruses, bacteria, and toxins as "criminals" being "routed" by the body's "police force.") Quite often, the analogies applied to the immune system derive, appropriately enough, from the battlefield, complete with allusions to "cellular foot soldiers," "biological arms factories," "mutinous macrophages," and "chemical warriors."

"The Wars Within" was how *National Geographic* recently headlined a lavishly illustrated article on the immune system that opened, "Besieged by a vast array of invisible enemies, the human body enlists a remarkably complex corps of internal bodyguards to battle the invaders."[1] In an article on AIDS published by the Baylor College of Medicine, a doctor likened the T-4 lymphocyte to "a traffic cop at a busy intersection," and the different types of cells to cars. "The T-4 lymphocytes regulate the flow of immunologic traffic," the doctor went on. "Take away the cops, and you have chaos. This is what happens in AIDS patients."[2]

This last analogy is, actually, quite accurate with regard to AIDS. It is easy to visualize the immune system as a place of heavy traffic, especially when an infection threatens; and, under ordinary circumstances, when all its components — all of its various watchdogs and biochemical neutralizing strategies — are working properly, the immune system is, truly, a bulwark against infection.

But the circumstances of a given infection can confound the body's defense mechanisms. For example, the number of germs or viruses that actually enter the body is an important factor in determining the severity of an infection: the larger the number of germs, the more severe the infection may be expected to be. Hordes of germs and viruses are also able to use certain counterstrategies that enable them to slip by the immune system. Moreover, the system itself depends heavily on an individual's physical characteristics and general fitness for its efficiency. Under the influences of age, gender, inadequate rest and nutrition, disease — such as flu, malaria, tuberculosis, even measles — or some environmental factor (such as humidity and temperature), the immune system can be temporarily weakened, opening the door to infections that other people would withstand. Generally, though, when adverse influences are resolved, the impaired immune system returns to normal. Such is not the case, however, with an AIDS infection. Not only does the virus take full advantage of all of the immune system's loopholes, but the immune deficiency it causes is permanent.

An AIDS infection begins when the virus enters the bloodstream of its victim, locks on to the receptor sites on the cells it chooses to infect, and, through some mechanism not yet fully understood, penetrates the cell membrane, losing its protective protein coating in the process. In about half an hour, the uncoated virus, now essentially a strand of RNA and a supply of reverse transcriptase, is floating about in the cytoplasm of the cell, the jellylike material that surrounds the nucleus. In this naked state, it is as dangerous as a stripped, live electrical wire. While still in the cytoplasm, the uncoated virus converts its RNA into double-stranded DNA, which then finds its way into the cell's nucleus, inserts itself into the chromosomes, and seizes control of the cellular machinery.

Once its RNA is translated into DNA and is nestled in the cellular chromosomes, the virus may hole up like that for weeks, months, or even years without causing any ill effects; this is the latent period, or so-called carrier state. Some men have been infected for at least five years without showing any signs of the disease. (Coming up with a clear estimate of how long someone has been infected is not always possible because of uncertainty over just when the virus was first acquired.)

Typically, the time between initial contact with the virus and seroconversion — the time when antibodies actually develop against the alien — is six to eight weeks. Most people who become infected show no symptoms. But if during this latent period some of those virus-infected T-cells find their way into someone else, the disease can be transferred.

Eventually, the genetic material in the cell may, under conditions still not fully understood, but perhaps influenced by any of a wide range of other infections, become activated. Once that happens, the steady process that leads to the end stages of infection by the AIDS virus begins. Under the direction of the viral DNA, the cell makes copies of the virus at an alarming rate, and these then bud from the cell's surface, usually taking a piece of it along and often killing the cell in the process — but not before releasing a whole new family of viruses, which go on to infect other cells. That is what occurs when a single cell is infected. But cells divide during the process of mitosis, a division designed to ensure that all the cells of an individual are genetically identical. In the case of an AIDS infection, that means genetically identical not only to the cell itself but to the viral DNA that has fitted itself into the cell's chromosomes. Now, each time an infected cell divides, the virus and its blueprint appear in the new cells, and the scenario is played out all over again when the virus is activated: under the sway of the viral genes, more and more AIDS viruses swarm out of the new cells, inserting themselves in other cells.

Under such an onslaught, large numbers of T-4 cells are overwhelmed. With so many of those control cells now lost, the chemical messages that signal the B-cells and killer cells to action are weakened, and the structured environment of the immune system breaks down. Antibody production by the B-cells drops; killer cells and macrophages lose their destructive power or have it lessened. Unable to get an immune response going, what remains of the defense system leaves the door open to ordinarily harmless germs that now have free rein to produce sometimes fatal diseases. Because the breakdown is fairly selective — that is, it affects components of the immune system that ward off parasites, fungal organisms, and other viruses — AIDS victims usually develop a range of unusual infections, while sometimes resisting some of the more common ones.

Once the AIDS virus is churning out copies of itself at an explosive rate, nothing seems to be able to stop it. Within two years of its damaging assaults on the immune system, most of its victims are dead, and only a few manage to hang on longer than three years. Ironically, people infected with the virus do make antibodies against some of the virus's protein (as the current antibody tests prove). But whether the response means anything has yet to be determined.

Generally, AIDS patients make antibodies against viral proteins embedded both in the virus's core and in its envelope during the early phases of the disease, when there are no clinical symptoms. (The core proteins do not appear to be as important to the antigen-antibody process as the envelope proteins, although, as we will see later, researchers who are trying to develop an AIDS vaccine are interested in what role they might play.) Later, as the disease worsens and the swollen lymph nodes, multiple infections, cancer, and nervous-system disorders begin to show up, the anti-envelope protein antibodies are still there, but those made against the core proteins have declined. The significance of this finding has yet to be established, but the bottom line with regard to antibody production is that it does not seem to offer much protection, if any, to someone infected by the virus.

Researchers have succeeded in destroying AIDS-infected T-4 cells in the laboratory with antibodies taken from AIDS patients, but it is apparently a different story in a victim's body: most of the AIDS-generated antibodies do not do the job they are supposed to do — that is, to inactivate or kill the virus — and the patients get sick, either immediately or eventually, despite their presence. Some people infected with the virus do seem to be free of clinical symptoms for some time, but others get sick and die in a fairly short time. This could mean either that the strength, or lack, of an immune response to the virus differs from patient to patient, or that the many AIDS virus strains that enter the body provoke individual, different responses.

That the HIV virus homes in on the T-4 cells is, of course, the reason for the "immune deficiency" part of the disease known as AIDS. But destruction of the immune system, clinicians and researchers now know, is but one of the manifestations of infection by the virus. Sometimes, the signs of such an infection — the neurological disorders, the opportunistic infections, and the cancers — can occur in the absence of any immune deficiency. That is why some doctors refer to an HIV epidemic, rather than an AIDS epidemic. (The disease known as AIDS — the end stage of infection with the AIDS virus — was defined as such for national reporting long before its cause was discovered, and because of that, the definition was far too narrow.)

There are, it now appears, plenty of cells other than the T-4 cells for the virus to choose to attack. Its list of targets has grown considerably, and now includes B-cells, macrophages, monocytes (large phagocytic white cells), nerve cells, and perhaps the killer T-cells — anything, it seems, that carries T-4 receptors on its surface, or some molecule resembling it.

But it is the AIDS virus's ability to infect the brain and produce serious neurological, motor, and psychological consequences that has emerged as a clear indication of the virus's versatility. Newborn babies infected with HIV seem to be especially vulnerable to brain infection by the virus, and approximately 70 percent of adult AIDS patients suffer from neuropsychiatric disorders, including depression, delirium, and a severe dementia that causes slurred speech, slowed movements, loss of memory, and psychosis. In addition, neurologists at the Johns Hopkins Medical Institutions have found that many patients also have peripheral neuropathies — painful numbness in one or more limbs, or weakness — which may mean that the virus settles in the peripheral nervous system as well as the brain.

Such findings do not bode well for treatment possibilities for

AIDS, because many drugs cannot breach the so-called blood-brain barrier, a sturdy, semipermeable membrane that effectively cuts off the brain from the rest of the body and prevents large molecules from reaching it. Hidden in such a sanctuary, the AIDS virus is free to sit still, yet dangerous, like a chemical time bomb, or to start up the same devastating, replicating process it does when it is in the immune cells.

When AIDS was first diagnosed in 1981, doctors believed that the unusually high incidence of neurological difficulties that had been turning up in patients with the disease were due to the stress of suffering from so devastating and fatal an illness. Later, they became aware that many of those same neurological ills were caused by secondary infections such as toxoplasmosis or herpes. But they still could not quite explain why other AIDS patients had equally severe neurological problems in the absence of those infections. Nor could they understand why some of the psychiatric disturbances seemed to be particularly severe, even in those patients who had no history of emotional illness. There was a clue, though: some of the psychiatric symptoms associated with AIDS emerged long before any physical signs — which is what would occur if the virus, which can hide in the bloodstream for years before it is activated and starts up the disease process, had a direct effect on the central nervous system.

The mystery appeared solved with the publication in *The Lancet* in 1985 of a paper by researchers from the University of California at San Francisco. The principal author, virologist Jay Levy (who had discovered one of the first AIDS viruses), reported that he had isolated the virus in samples from the cerebrospinal fluid and the brain tissues of homosexuals suffering from AIDS and its underlying neurological problems. Said Levy: "The results suggest that ARV [Levy's designation for the virus] could be the cause of the neurological syndromes in AIDS patients, and indicate that the virus can infect cells other than T-lymphocytes."[3]

But what brain cell types did the virus invade? Since the AIDS virus was showing signs of a similarity to the subfamily of lentiviruses, did it also attack, as the visna and caprine viruses did, the large white cells, the macrophages and the monocytes?

After Levy's report was published, neurologist Sid Houff of the National Institute of Neurological and Communicative Disorders and Stroke said that he was not surprised by Levy's findings since so many of the AIDS patients were suffering from a neurological problem. He indicated that T-4 cells would seem to be the logical victims, because they are found in the brain as well as in other parts of the body. But Houff refused at the time to rule out the possibility that other types of brain cells — such as glial cells, which support neurons (nerve cells) and provide their nourishment, and macrophages — were also targets. His reasoning was sound: brain cells have many of the chemical markers found on the surface of lymphocytes, and these markers might be the ones most easily recognized by the AIDS virus.

By mid-1986, scientists had at least partially resolved the question of which cells in the brain the AIDS virus seemed to concentrate on. Examining the autopsied brains of twelve AIDS patients, all of which were mildly inflamed, Clayton Wiley of the University of California at San Diego and his colleagues found the virus in nine. The cells that were most commonly infected turned out to be macrophages, monocytes, and the endothelial cells, the ones that form the inner lining of body cavities, blood vessels, lymph channels — and the brain capillaries. Only one brain showed evidence of neuronal or glial infection, but that one, too, had more infected macrophages and giant cells than cells that appeared to be neurons or glia. Moreover, Wiley found, the AIDS virus seemed to be rather selective for the brain's endothelial cells, because that type of cell was not infected elsewhere in the body.[4]

Other researchers who have found the virus in the brains of AIDS patients speculate that perhaps the virus first infects macrophages somewhere else in the victim's body; these then migrate to the brain, effectively seeding it. If that is true, it could explain both how the virus gets from the blood to the brain to cause disease there and how it manages to lie dormant for so long.

It has been known for some time that the virus "hides" somewhere in the body when it is not infecting T-4 cells. Scientists know this because they have only rarely been able to find the virus in circulating T-4 cells, probably because the cells die so fast. Because macrophages roam at will from blood to tissues throughout the body and can carry the virus without being killed by it, it has been theorized that the scavenger cells harbor the virus before passing it to the T-4 cells. (The Langerhans' cells, immune system cells found in the outer layer of the skin, are also suspect as the reservoir in which the AIDS virus hides until it is time to infect. These cells, which carry the T-4 marker, are known to pick up a foreign antigen and pass it on to the T-cells, and have turned up in skin samples from patients with AIDS and ARC.)

What happens once the AIDS virus finds its way into the brain is still conjecture. Wiley's study found that although AIDS patients suffer severe neurological disturbances, their expected brain tissue abnormalities were surprisingly mild, and there was rarely, if ever, direct infection of nerve cells. But Wiley and his associates speculated that the virus causes brain damage indirectly, by producing edema in the brain, an excessive accumulation of fluids, much as radiation treatment causes edema in some cancer patients; the swelling, in turn, can cause generalized damage in the brain, disrupting its delicate chemical communications system to produce a number of neurological deficits, including dementia. As Wiley explained it: "Something elicits the migration of macrophages into the brain and in deep white matter there is swelling."[5] Speculation is that infected macrophages secrete soluble substances that cause edema or perhaps other forms of tissue damage. Once the endothelial cells in the brain capillaries are infected, they could leak, thus compounding the edema problem and shifting the brain's crucial balances and concentrations of ions and crucial electrolytes such as potassium, sodium, and chlorides. If such hypotheses are true, they could mean that it may not be necessary for the AIDS virus to infect large numbers of neurons to play havoc with brain function.[6]

Generally speaking, though, the chance of developing an AIDS infection, and the severity of the various other illnesses observed after infection by the AIDS virus, are probably related to the intensity of viral replication — that is, to how much virus is being turned loose in the immune system, and how many T-cells are infected. Thus, a small dose of the AIDS virus would probably not be enough to infect a person because the body's defenses would be able to handle it. What actually constitutes a "small" dose and whether that term even means anything in virology are still unclear, however; one man's small dose under the wrong conditions could be another man's disaster.

Researchers still do not know how much of the virus has to get into the body to cause an infection, but the fact that lab and health care workers who accidentally stick themselves with HIV-contaminated needles rarely contract AIDS, while promiscuous homosexuals and IV-drug abusers are in grave danger of doing so, is pretty good proof that it takes a fairly large dose. I asked Dr. Albert Sabin, who developed the oral polio vaccine and recently served as an NIH consultant, whether a single virus could cause either polio or AIDS. His reponse:

> Rarely. There was a time when dysentery was a serious disease in the U.S., and they wouldn't discharge a patient from the hospital and let him go back to work as long as his stools had some dysentery bacillus. Later, it was proved that small amounts of dysentery bacillus did not transmit infection, and they could be there for years and years and the person would be harmless to others.
>
> It's the same with polio. It's not a question of one particle. It's not just that virus is present, virus is absent. That's not good enough. From everything we know about infectious diseases, it's not just the presence, it's the quantity, and what happens where it multiplies.
>
> Surely a trace of the virus somewhere, in tears, saliva, the vaginal mucosa, doesn't mean the disease is transmitted that way. You have to ask how much of the virus is there, and whether it's really associated with cells, or just free. I've been in the field for a half-century, and believe me, we've been through this with all diseases.

While that speaks against acquiring AIDS through casual contact, it does not, of course, strip the virus of the formidable power that it does have. The process by which it replicates, once it is started up, is most efficient, and frighteningly so. And here appears to be one of those times when this virus does seem to have a mind of its own: some intricate inner mechanism that enables it to direct the rapid-fire multiplication of itself — 100 times faster than other retroviruses — that has become one of its hallmarks; some master chemical switch, perhaps, that makes it the most complex virus of its class.

There is, it turns out, such a switch in the core of the virus. Discovered only in 1986, it is the gene known as tat-III, and it directs one of the most powerful biological amplifiers ever found. Standing for "trans-acting transcription regulation," tat-III — whose discovery was a collaborative effort by Gallo's team and that of William Haseltine, a pathologist and AIDS researcher at Boston's Dana-Farber Cancer Institute and Harvard Medical School — provided the first clue to the mechanism by which the AIDS virus may transform cells and thus cause wild proliferation of the virus and destruction of the immune system defenses.

Under the general rules of molecular biology, genetic information flows from DNA to messenger RNA in the process known as transcription. Sometimes RNA is the gene's final product, and other times it is a protein product; this process, from RNA to proteins, is called translation. Thus, the regulation of RNA production is the most commonly recognized growth-control mechanism.

In the case of the AIDS virus, its tat-III gene produces a protein (called the trans-activator) that greatly increases the ability of the infected cells to produce new virus particles. This trans-activator protein, Haseltine and his colleagues had demonstrated earlier, enabled the HTLV-I and HTLV-II retroviruses to produce a 100-fold increase in the production of proteins from viral DNA. Later, they discovered that trans-activation also took place in HTLV-III, but at a much higher rate. As Haseltine put it: "In HTLV-III, trans-activation appears to increase translation 1,000- or in some cases 5,000-fold. If HTLV-I and HTLV-II could be said to make virus particles at the rate of piston engines, HTLV-III's replication system could be compared to a jet engine."[7] The reason behind the different rates, it turned out, was the tat-III gene, which, although it has analogues in HTLV-I and HTLV-II, apparently works in other ways.

In their early studies of HTLV-III trans-activation, Haseltine's team assumed that overproduction of viral proteins would be the result of a permutation of the transcription process that caused overproduction of viral RNA; this had been shown to be the case in most regulated genes, and was also what happened in both HTLV-I and HTLV-II. That is, in those two virus strains, the increase in gene expression resulted from an increase in the rate in which RNA was transcribed from viral DNA. It turned out, however, to be a different story with the AIDS virus, HTLV-III. Instead of regulating the amount of RNA, the interim step in the production of protein, the AIDS virus circumvented that step, speeding up production of the virus-making trans-activator protein by directly increasing translation of messenger RNA into protein.

"The major impact of this discovery is on our thinking," said Haseltine, who believes that the newly discovered mechanism may be used by other genes as well as those in viruses. "This enables us to reevaluate the possibilities of gene regulation in mammalian cells. The three to four order of magnitude increase in translation efficiency observed here opens the question of what we really know about the step of protein synthesis that lies between export from the nucleus and initiation of protein synthesis."[8]

But beyond the purely basic science of learning more about gene control, and beyond pinpointing the mechanism by which the AIDS virus extends its life cycle, there are some practical applications for tat-III. One is that the same mechanism can be harnessed to produce high levels of proteins in animal cells — cells in which many of the biological products potentially useful as pharmaceuticals are now made. But such current methods of protein manufacture are cumbersome and inefficient, and although bacteria and yeast cells are often used to produce some biological products, they do not modify the finished proteins in the way that animal cells do. Haseltine's group successfully introduced the tat-III gene into a number of different cell lines, including several suitable for producing useful proteins, and achieved enormous overproduction. Moreover, some of these proteins are selected from the AIDS virus itself, including the envelope glycoprotein antigen thought to be the most important part of the virus for vaccine research. The discovery of tat-III also provides AIDS researchers with an important attack point in the virus: if drugs could be designed to interfere with the master switch, the spread of the virus could perhaps be stopped.

The tat-III gene — and another regulatory gene, called art, discovered by Haseltine's group — may also explain the slow pattern of many AIDS infections and the way the virus often lies still in the T-cells. During this latent state, viral RNA may be produced, but no new virus particles. When the T-cells are activated, perhaps by some other infection, so, too, are the tat-III and art genes, and these produce the cell-killing virus particles.

But for all of this apparent certainty about what makes the AIDS virus such a swift-replicating killer — and thus such a fearful opponent — a central question has yet to be fully resolved: How does the virus actually go about killing the T-cells? The question is no mere academic exercise, for until researchers can identify the critical stages in the cell-destroying process and learn more about the way the AIDS virus depletes the immune system of its helper cells, they can forget about developing a vaccine or anti-AIDS drugs.

The high rate of trans-activation in the AIDS virus may account at least partly for the virus's rapid cell-killing activity, but, at this writing at least, the exact role that tat-III plays in that destruction is still unclear. (When the gene is snipped out of the virus, it does not kill T-cells and does not reproduce.) The most popular generally stated hypothesis is that after the virus commandeers the host cell to produce new viruses, it ultimately works the host cell to death in the process.

Gallo has proposed that the virus kills T-4 cells by turning on the cells' genes that enable the cells to complete their life cycle. With its own genes part of the DNA of the T-4 cells, and mimicking the cells' own regulator genes, the T-4 cell bursts into action, producing all the proteins it is meant to produce only when an immune response is stimulated. The cells then die prematurely.[9]

Another possibility is that helper T-cells infected with the

AIDS virus fuse with healthy, uninfected cells to form giant agglomerates that produce large quantities of the virus and then die. According to pathologist Edgar Engleman, whose team at the Stanford Medical Center has proposed the theory, a single infected cell can fuse with several healthy cells, sopping them up and killing them. Thus, the disappearance of helper cells into dying giant cells could contribute to the collapse of immune defenses that characterizes AIDS.[10] The fusion theory also means that the AIDS virus might be able to avoid the bloodstream and, hence, the surveillance cells of the immune system: when the cell it has infected joins with another, the virus can glide through — under cover, as it were — into the other cell, without having to risk going out into a hostile environment.

Still another possibility is put forth by Pasteur scientists. They suspect that the T-4 cells are killed by the body's own killer T-cells in one of those odd twists in the immune response, called autoimmunity, by which the body fights off its own components, treating them as nonself. The autoimmune response in AIDS, when there is one, occurs because the T-4 cells carry foreign proteins in their cell membranes; the killer T-cells, regarding that situation as an invasion by foreign substances, turn on the T-4 cells and destroy them in a case of mistaken identity.

It is interesting to note that a clue to how the AIDS virus destroys cells may come not only from the killer itself but from a more benign cousin, a newfound virus that is closely related to the AIDS virus but that appears to be harmless. Called HTLV-IV by Max Essex, whose team discovered it in the blood of healthy people in Senegal (and, as expected, called LAV-II by the Pasteur team, which simultaneously reported finding one like it, also in West Africans, but in individuals with symptoms of AIDS), the new agent is structurally similar to HTLV-III, and to STLV-III, the virus found in the green monkeys.

"We believe it is a 'missing link' virus somewhere between the virus that infects healthy African greens, and the virus infecting AIDS patients in Africa and in the U.S.," Essex said in announcing the discovery. Because of the similarity, isolation of HTLV-IV might well provide more clues to the origins of the human AIDS virus, but right now it is what sets HTLV-IV apart from its lethal relative that is more important than its place on the evolutionary chart from monkey to man, for comparisons between the two may eventually lead to the answer to the AIDS virus's destructiveness. The main difference between the two strains is that in lab cultures HTLV-IV infects the same T-cells that the AIDS virus does, but without the dramatic killing action. Also, none of the more than fifty people infected with HTLV-IV have developed any AIDS symptoms, thirty of them after more than a year's follow-up. "Only two things can be happening here," Essex observed. "Either these people have a better immune response, or the virus isn't as deadly. Probably it's a combination of the two."[11]

The relationship between HTLV-IV and the French virus, LAV-II, is not clear at this writing. In November 1986, Luc Montagnier reported that though his new virus was at first thought to cause AIDS only rarely, new evidence suggested that LAV-II may be as deadly as the original AIDS virus and that it was, indeed, a main cause of the disease in West Africa and perhaps in several Western European countries as well. "We are just at the beginning of the spread of a new virus," he commented. "It is unavoidable at some time that LAV-II will reach the United States."[12]

In May 1987, new studies by Dr. François Clavel of the Institut Pasteur appeared to confirm the concerns about LAV-II (now known as HIV-II): it had turned up in 30 people, most of them in western Africa; 17 had AIDS, and the rest had AIDS-related complex or no symptoms. None had been infected with the virus known to cause AIDS. Reported the researchers in the *New England Journal of Medicine:* "It appears that HIV-2, a virus related to but distinct from HIV-1, is the cause of AIDS in some West Africans and that a new AIDS epidemic is possible, but not yet documented, in West Africa. The precise extent of the spread of the virus toward other areas, including other parts of Africa and Europe, will have to be assessed by large-scale prospective seroepidemiologic studies."[13]

An interesting sidelight to the HIV-II discovery is that the virus could conceivably be a natural vaccine, one that protects those it infects against the real AIDS virus, in much the same way that people with cowpox are invulnerable to smallpox. When scientists went back and examined blood samples taken some years ago in Senegal, they found indications that HIV-II was present there for at least ten years. What makes that finding significant is that although AIDS is epidemic in central Africa, few cases have been reported in Senegal.

Whether HIV-II does serve as nature's vaccine against AIDS has yet to be determined, but Essex's group is watching female prostitutes in Senegal, many of whom have HIV-II infection, and who are likely to be exposed to the AIDS virus as well since it appears to be spreading from central Africa. If those people infected with HIV-II (who do not lose any T-4 cells when infected with the virus strain) show losses in their T-4 cells after exposure to the AIDS virus, then there is no protection; if they do not lose T-4 cells, that would be a fairly good indication that HIV-II is having some protective effect. The same sort of watch-dogging is going on in the laboratory. By adding AIDS virus to cells infected with HIV-II, the researchers hope to find out what, if anything, the AIDS virus does to those cells.

If HIV-II does set up some barrier against the AIDS virus, it might also lend credence to suggestions that have been made recently by some scientists that once a particular strain of the AIDS virus gets a hold in the body, it effectively bars all other AIDS virus variants from getting in. The rationale behind this comes from analyzing viral genes in AIDS-infected persons and comparing them with one another. In many instances, the strains found in one individual's body were far more similar to each other than they were when matched against those of another person. If, as is true of many AIDS victims, each person had had multiple sex partners, then it should follow that all of these people would carry a number of different viruses because they had presumably been exposed to so many strains. But since this apparently is not always the case, and patients did not appear to have multiple virus strains in their bodies, the first AIDS virus that gained entry, according to the theory, propagated its own family, complete with minor variations, while setting up some sort of defense against others that might try to infect.

Getting at the truth of that, however, will take some time

since there is not, at this moment certainly, even the hint of a clue to the mechanism. At a conference on AIDS held in Paris in June of 1986, Gallo presented evidence that the AIDS virus differs not only between and within individuals over time, but also in the different parts of the body it chooses to infect. For instance, the virus that infects brain cells seems to be more efficient at infecting brain cells than the variant that hits T-4 cells — a phenomenon that indicates some sort of viral natural selection. Experiments in Sweden showed similar selectivity: virus removed from late-stage AIDS patients appeared to be better at infecting T-4 cells than viruses taken from patients in the earlier stages of the disease. According to Gallo, not one but several strains of AIDS virus infect a person, and these strains fit the best environmental conditions in various parts of the body; at any one time, one viral strain might dominate, but there are always others there to take its place.[14] Indeed, researchers believe that many other new AIDS viruses besides HIV-II may surface. If that is the case, the search for drugs to combat them and a vaccine to prevent an infection by them will be all the harder.

6

How Did the Virus Go from Monkeys to Humans?

DETERMINING EXACTLY HOW the AIDS virus causes an infection is not the only thorny question facing researchers today. Another nettling one is how did the virus get from monkeys to humans, and from Africa to the Western world? Again, speculation abounds.

When I put the question to Harvard's William Haseltine, he explained it this way:

> Human, and human parasite, evolution occurred over hundreds of thousands, millions, of years. Therefore, a lot of parasites have adapted to us and our predecessors — microbial parasites, viruses, worms. Even today, in Africa, there's a war being fought between us and our parasites, a war that keeps human beings out of certain reaches of the continent. The tsetse fly is back, and Africa is clear of people in the areas where it lives. There are places where malaria is so endemic that a human can't go there without getting malaria.
>
> Now, generally, we've adapted to the wide variety of parasites pretty well. We've had to, or we wouldn't have survived. And monkeys have had to, too. But all it takes is the transmission of one of those microbial parasites that's become well-adapted to one of our relatives, in this case the green monkey. It gets into us, and we researchers see it in five to ten years. Bingo, that's it. We humans have freed ourselves from those African parasites, more or less,

by our migrations. But they're still there, and they're highly evolved for entry into our species.

But once the simian virus jumped the species line, how did it get into humans to cause AIDS? Here, hard science gives way to speculation. Parasitologists are fully aware, of course, that disease can easily be transmitted to humans by an animal's bites, or even by simple contact with their infected secretions. The list is familiar, and almost endless: malaria, rat-bite fever, rabies, typhus, bubonic plague, Lyme disease, encephalitis, and cat-scratch disease, to name but a few. The AIDS virus, too, might well have been passed to humans in the same way that many other diseases are, through bites and scratches.

That the virus was plentiful in the African AIDS belt was a given: Max Essex, with Phyllis Kanki, a postdoctoral fellow at Harvard, had found that one-half to two-thirds of the green monkeys were infected with the simian analogue of the AIDS virus. It thus was not difficult to extrapolate from that and come up with a reasonable answer as to how the virus got into humans. The animals forage in garbage dumps and, when people try to chase them away, they sometimes fight back by biting and scratching. The natives also sell the monkeys, and sometimes eat their flesh.

Such close contact with infected animals explained how the mutated AIDS virus may have found its way into human beings, but how did it get out of Africa? No one knows for sure, but it goes without saying that it had to get out some way. HTLV-I, for example, according to Gallo, occurs precisely in areas of southern Japan where Portuguese explorers, slave traders, and commercial agents made their initial contacts. "The Portuguese established themselves throughout the southern portion of Japan and their influence and contact with the Japanese became frequent," he wrote recently in the British journal *Nature*.

It is known that the Portuguese took Africans with them to Japan. The Africans' presence can be seen in Portuguese pictorial records known as Nanban-Byobu, where the artist depicted Portuguese, Japanese and Africans together. Further, it is believed that the Portuguese came with African monkeys. The Japanese word for monkey, amakawa, is thought to be derived from the Portuguese word macaco, also meaning monkey. Recently [other researchers] supported this conclusion by demonstrating that the proportion of HTLV-I disease was correlated with the incidence of Japanese Catholics, again consistent with this hypothesis.[1]

The AIDS virus, it has been suggested, may have come by way of Haiti. During the mid-1970s, thousands of people participated in cultural exchanges between the French-speaking populations of Zaire and the Caribbean island. AIDS eventually could have been carried from Haiti to New York by American homosexuals, for whom the island had become a popular vacation spot. It then could have moved quickly from the United States to other parts of the world, where — like the smallpox brought to vulnerable American Indians by Europeans in the sixteenth century, and the deadly measles epidemic visited upon the Fiji Islanders in the 1800s — it settled in and began its work of infecting the relatively closed homosexual and drug-abusing communities, in which the practices essential to infection were ideal.

"Although the virus causing AIDS is surely American by adoption, not by birth, the epidemic is indeed all-American in its initial dissemination," observed June Osborn, dean of the University of Michigan School of Public Health and a professor of epidemiology.

Most of the rest of the world is catching up with us, with a lag time of two or three years, but the exportations from the United States are easily tracked. We are indeed one world in operational — if not in peaceful — terms. A recent paper from Japan, for instance, documented the absence of [the AIDS virus] antibody from a number of Japanese groups, including homosexuals, but reported 27 percent seropositivity among patients with hemophilia, which was directly related to the American source of [various blood] factors used to treat them. The introduction of AIDS into Denmark and Australia was readily traceable to the return of homosexual men from vacations in New

York and San Francisco. Even the presence of the poor Haitians in the high-risk category may reflect the penchant of American homosexual men for vacationing in Haiti, coupled with the dire poverty that makes prostitution a frequent means of subsistence survival for Haitian adolescents of either sex. A recent analysis of the distribution of infection in Haiti showed a typical frequency of [the AIDS virus] antibody in the general population, contrasting with a markedly higher frequency in areas known to be centers for prostitution, male and female alike.[2]

7

How Contagious Is AIDS?

> I may be told by some that men may contract syphilis by
> sitting in a public privy; to this I can only answer that I
> have never witnessed a single instance; nor did the late
> Mr. Obre, who had been for many years extensively en-
> gaged in treating venereal disease; for on asking him if he
> believed that the disease was propagated in this manner,
> he shrewdly answered, that it sometimes was the manner
> in which married men contracted it, but unmarried men
> never caught it in this manner.
>
> — *Abraham Colles*

AIDS BECAME A NATIONAL OBSESSION almost from the moment
it surfaced and began wrecking the immune systems of its victims. Dr. George Galasso, a member of the NIH's task force
on the disease, told me:

> The reason people are so terribly concerned over AIDS
> is that any time there's a new disease they don't under-
> stand, they're afraid it's going to grow bigger. Legion-
> naires' disease is an example, and you remember what
> happened there? It was a big scare for a few months, but
> the threat didn't last. We found out what it was and we
> were able to treat it.
>
> But with AIDS, we haven't leveled off yet. Initially, it
> was in populations. Now some people are more concerned
> because we're seeing it more as a heterosexual problem.
> We know the virus is changing. Is the population at risk

going to keep changing? Is the infection going to worsen? We don't know.

Since that statement was made, AIDS seems to have taken a turn for the worse. Its current death toll is awesome, especially considering that only sixteen cases had been reported between January and June of 1981. As many as 1.5 million Americans are now believed infected, although several specialists argue that the official estimates are greatly underestimated, perhaps by as much as a half. In New York, the hardest-hit city, one out of every fifteen persons carries the virus, and perhaps between one-fifth and one-half of those will contract the disease itself. That prediction may be conservative: in December 1986, a team of West German scientists projected that three-fourths of those infected with the virus would progress to the final, and fatal, stages of the disease within seven years. At this writing, some 50,000 cases have shown up in 112 countries, not including some hard-hit African nations; but officials of the World Health Organization estimate the real figure is about 100,000. As many as 10 million people might be infected, but are still without symptoms.

Latin American nations recently reported significant, steady rises in the number of their cases, a situation that is reminiscent of what happened in the United States and Africa a few years back. In Brazil, for example, reported cases totaled only 6 in 1982; but in 1984, 138 were recorded, and near the end of 1986, the total stood at more than 800.

There is still grimmer news. The U.S. Public Health Service, in its latest estimate of where the disease is going here, said this:

- By the end of 1991, some 270,000 AIDS cases will have occurred in the United States, with more than 74,000 occurring in that year alone.
- By the time 1991 ends, 179,000 people will have died of AIDS in the United States — 54,000 of those deaths occurring in that year (more than all the Americans who died in the entire Vietnam War).
- New AIDS cases spread through heterosexual contact

will increase from 1,100 in 1986 to nearly 7,000 in 1991.

• Pediatric AIDS cases will increase tenfold over the next four years, to more than 3,000 cumulative cases by the end of 1991.

Said the Institute of Medicine of the National Academy of Sciences in a 1986 report on the AIDS crisis: "In view of the numbers of people now infected, it is extremely unlikely that the rising incidence of AIDS will soon reverse itself. Disease and death resulting from [AIDS-virus] infection are likely to be increasing five to 10 years from now and probably into the next century."[1]

In light of such stark reality, America's, and the world's, dread of this new disease is understandable. AIDS does show signs of developing into a health disaster that poses enormous challenges for those who hope to eradicate it; and it carries with it, at this stage at least, an automatic sentence of death, with the dubious consolation for some of only a stay of execution. In a sense, then, it is much like bubonic plague, the Black Death that ravaged Europe and large parts of the world during the Middle Ages and later. There are even gruesome similarities in some of the symptoms. Plague victims develop fevers, weakness, glandular swellings, central-nervous-system disturbances, dark spots or patches on the skin, or perhaps a pneumonic form of the disease that congests the lungs.

But the resemblance of AIDS to the Black Death, probably the most virulent of the human infectious diseases, must end there. For one thing, plague is caused by a bacterium, and it is primarily a disease of rodents that is transmitted to humans by fleas that have bitten infected animals. Moreover, the infection may be carried in the air, in food, and in water, and the disease is, thus, spread more readily than AIDS. Then there are the numbers of those struck down by the Black Death, which alone should dismiss any comparison to AIDS as purely rhetorical. Plague carried enormous mortality, wiping out at least a third of the population of Europe, perhaps 25 million people. In A.D. 78, plague is said to have killed 10,000 people in one day alone in Rome; in 1348, 90,000 died in Germany; in 1611, 200,000 in

Constantinople. Great Britain, which went through a succession of plague outbreaks, lost one in three of its population.

It is, perhaps, unwise to invoke such mortality statistics to establish where AIDS really fits in the spectrum of humanity's afflictions, since even a single death because of a disease or accident may be viewed as tragic. But the fact remains that the death toll from AIDS, as dreadful as it is, covers six years, not a few months. Those figures, and even the ones projected for 1991, pale beside those of a disease far more familiar to us than plague, or AIDS: cancer, which can strike anyone, in or out of so-called risk groups, and will kill an estimated 472,000 Americans this year alone. There is also measles, a viral disease; it not only spreads far more easily than AIDS, but kills infinitely more people — 2 million children a year, most of them in Africa and Latin America. A half-million more die annually from tuberculosis, a far more lethal disease than AIDS, and one that was responsible for one-fifth to one-quarter of all deaths in the industrial world in the nineteenth century. Around the turn of the century, it killed as many as 150,000 Americans a year.

Moreover, someone said recently, AIDS is not the only sexually transmitted disease that kills; gonorrhea and chlamydia, venereal diseases that infect some 6 million Americans every year, are responsible for around half of the 75,000 ectopic pregnancies each year, anomalies that kill the fetus and can cause maternal death. Congenital syphilis, again on the rise, kills infants, as does herpes.[2]

So, as calamitous and as frightening as AIDS is, there is simply no comparison between it and some of these other afflictions. AIDS is not even a single disease, as we have seen. It is a syndrome: a group of symptoms and diseases, opportunistic infections that kill because the AIDS virus has weakened the body's immune system, or because the immune system was feeble to begin with. And the rate of the killing depends on the diseases involved; some of them, such as pneumocystis pneumonia, kill more often than others, such as Kaposi's sarcoma.

Moreover, despite the authoritative ring to the statements of some researchers and epidemiologists, no one really knows where AIDS is going — no more than anyone can say what other diseases will actually become epidemic or pandemic, or which ones will strike cyclically, or which ones will not find populations that become genetically resistant to their pathogens. Researchers at this time do not even know how the AIDS virus goes about killing the cells it infects, or which infected individuals will eventually develop, and succumb to, the disease. With such important questions still to be answered, to tell the world, based on the relatively few cases that seem to have broken out of the narrow confines of the AIDS boundaries in the United States, that "heterosexual AIDS cases are doubling every six months," as one recent community health specialist had it, is license of an incredibly broad nature.

The continual and strident barrage of scary rhetoric from some scientists, public health specialists, and elements of the media who merely dutifully report what they hear — the ominous word that AIDS is everywhere, that everyone is at risk — has also helped inflate the AIDS issue. "We as a society are faced with a major peril to our entire species," one pathologist told me. "We have not seen anything that we can't control except nuclear bombs that's of this magnitude. We've got big problems."

Such talk has dulled the repeated assertions of other, more attuned, specialists, who point out that we are talking about a disease that has, at most, infected only 1 percent or so of the U.S. population; that only a tiny fraction of that 1 percent has actually gone on to full-blown AIDS; that fairly large quantities of AIDS virus are probably needed to pass on the disease; that the routes the virus chooses to invade a human being are quite limited; that the available evidence only suggests, but does not prove, that heterosexual transmission is becoming more common; that it is highly improbable that exposure to toilet seats, drinking glasses, doorknobs, shower stalls, or food touched by an AIDS victim, or to sneezes, coughs, saliva, tears, or sweat of a victim, will result in an infection, and that in fact nobody is known to have contracted it that way; that AIDS is a blood-borne disease that in most cases strikes and will continue to strike (1) homosexual and bisexual males who have been the receptive partners in anal sex, (2) intravenous-drug abusers who share contaminated needles, and (3) children unfortunate enough to be born to infected mothers, many of whom will have acquired the disease through sharing of needles, or, on rarer occasions, through conventional sex with an infected partner, or, on still fewer occasions (because the nation's blood supply is now safer), through a tainted blood transfusion.

In 1986, Dr. Albert Sabin put the AIDS issue in what many feel is its proper perspective. "AIDS is obviously an important new disease," he told me, "but — and that's a big 'but' — there's been created around it a hysteria which, in my judgment, is unfounded. AIDS, after all, is and remains a disease of a limited portion of the population, and there is no indication that it is going to involve the general population. I think AIDS is an interesting disease, but its relative public health importance is minuscule by comparison with many far more serious problems that make it look like a speck floating on the ocean. It has been blown out of all proportion."

Nevertheless, many individuals — especially Americans, who seem to be particularly susceptible to germ phobia — still hold the irrational notion that the AIDS virus is a superagent, an Andromeda strain with the transmission efficiency of the common cold that is bound to strike down everybody in its path. That is why fourteen prospective jurors in Stamford, Connecticut, asked to be excused from a murder case after sheriff's deputies wearing rubber gloves escorted in the accused, who had been diagnosed as having AIDS. That is why the only empty seat in a crowded New York City subway car was the one on which someone had spray-painted, "Did an AIDS patient sit here last?" And that is why the Episcopal bishop of California issued a pastoral letter addressing parishioners' fear of drinking communion wine from a common cup. And why a judge in Indianapolis forbade a divorced father infected with the AIDS virus from seeing his two-year-old daughter, and why two inmates of a Florida prison put blood serum from an AIDS patient into a correction officer's coffee cup, and why a California congressman said he would introduce legislation making it a federal crime for AIDS victims and those infected with the virus to have sex or kiss.

That is also why the Justice Department decided that employers may fire workers with AIDS; why kids with AIDS in Queens, New York, and Kokomo, Indiana, were barred from attending school; why doctors are listing the cause of death from AIDS as "respiratory failure"; why neighbors of a Santa Monica, California, woman whose husband died of AIDS slipped notes under her apartment door that read, "Move," and "People like you shouldn't live around normal people"; why thirty-nine sanitation workers refused to take their trucks from a Harlem garage in protest over the presence of a fellow employee who had AIDS; and why a telephone lineman in Massachusetts who worked with an employee with AIDS said, "I've got three kids and I'm afraid of what I don't know and what the doctors don't know."

There is homophobia, too, in the AIDS-plague mentality. It is evident in the uneasy feeling some people express when they are served by an apparently gay waiter, or, as happened during a city council election in New York City, when they refuse to accept a gay candidate's campaign literature; it is there in the incredibly crude and cruel comments that AIDS stands for "Another Infected Dick Sucker" and that *gay* stands for "Got AIDS Yet?"; and it is there when political extremist Lyndon LaRouche and his followers organize a Prevent AIDS Now Initiative Committee (PANIC) and call for quarantining AIDS carriers; and when the Vatican announces that gay advocates seem to be undeterred by the realization that "homosexuality may seriously threaten the lives and well-being of a large number of people"; and when gay activists charge before a House Judiciary Subcommittee that physical attacks on homosexuals, including homicides, have increased over the last three years; and when the U.S. Supreme Court rules that the Constitution does not give consenting adults the right to engage in private homosexual activity, and upholds a Georgia antisodomy law that prohibits oral and anal sex and makes those acts punishable by a prison term of up to twenty years.

Often downplayed in all of this heated arguing over the disease and the groups it afflicts — perhaps because doing so tends to diminish the gravity of the disease when it might be expedient to keep up the drumfire — are the definitions of infectious communicable diseases and contagious ones. If the descriptions are not ignored, they are quite often confused. An infectious disease is simply one that is capable of causing an infection. *Contagious* is often used to measure how easily an infectious disease is spread — whether it can be "caught." Measles, for example, is both infectious and very contagious, readily transmitted by airborne droplets of sputum, by direct contact with nasal or throat secretions or the urine of infected persons, and by such things as handkerchiefs, napkins, and sheets freshly soiled with nose and mouth secretions. Malaria, on the other hand, is transmitted by mosquitoes, often over great distances, and is infectious; but it is by no means contagious.

Based on what is now known about the AIDS virus, its modes of transmission, and its steady, predictable pattern of infectiveness, it can be said — and said without minimizing the wide range of the disease it causes, the number of victims it has claimed, or its virulence — that the AIDS virus is not as powerful as the public seems to believe, and that it is not very contagious, meaning it does not spread easily at all. (Robert Gallo has been known to take the virus home in a flask, and keep it in his refrigerator.)

Look at it this way: If you draw 1 cubic centimeter of blood, about enough to fill an eyedropper, from a person who is infected with the tenacious and widespread virus that causes hepatitis B (HBV), put it into a swimming pool containing 24,000 gallons of water, extract 1 cubic centimeter of water from the pool, and inject it into a chimpanzee, there will be enough virus in the shot to infect the chimp. But if you put the same amount of blood from someone who is infected with the AIDS virus into the pool, if the chlorine in the water did not kill the virus (which it almost certainly would), the virus would not infect a chimp — or a human being. Even if you diluted the virus in only a quart of water, the chances of giving a chimp AIDS with a 1cc shot of that water would be about one in ten.

Hepatitis B was used in the above example because the virus that causes the disease is the agent most often compared to the AIDS virus. Both are transmitted through sexual contact, exposure to contaminated blood or blood products, and perinatally, from infected mothers to their babies. Neither virus has been shown to be transmitted by casual contact in the workplace, through tainted food or water, ventilation systems, telephones, drinking fountains, or fecal contact. Thus, much that has been learned about how to lower the risk of acquiring a hepatitis infection can be applied to AIDS.

But, as with bubonic plague, there are vast gaps between the two diseases. Hepatitis B is by far more widespread, and much more easily acquired, than AIDS. Hepatitis B, in fact, is fast becoming the world's leading infectious killer, with conservative estimates indicating that there are more than a billion people infected throughout the world — 200 million as chronic carriers of the virus (which means they can pass it on to someone else) — 50 million new infections every year, and more than 2 million deaths a year. Some 200,000 cases a year occur in the United States. Unlike AIDS, hepatitis B is highly endemic in places like the People's Republic of China (500,000 to 1 million new cases every year) and Southeast Asia, where between 70 percent and 95 percent of the adult population will show signs in the blood of having been exposed to the disease; as many as 15 percent of the population in these areas can be carriers of the virus. Even eastern Europe, the Soviet Union, and the Middle East, thus far spared from AIDS, are endemic areas for hepatitis B: between 20 percent and 55 percent of the adult population has been exposed, and 2 percent to 7 percent are carriers.[3]

But hepatitis B is not only more prevalent than AIDS; it is, as the swimming-pool example demonstrates, much more potent. Moreover, concentrations of HBV in the blood of carriers are much higher compared with AIDS. Further proof of their relative potency comes from studies of those who work in health care settings, where the risk of acquiring an HBV infection following an accidental needle-stick from a carrier ranges from 6 percent to 30 percent. This is far in excess of the risk of an AIDS-virus infection after a similar accident, which is, according to the CDC, less than 1 percent.

In May 1987, three hospital workers, none of whom belonged to any high-risk group, tested positive for the AIDS virus after their skin was briefly exposed to infected blood. It was the first documented spread of the virus to health workers that did not involve a needle-stick or prolonged exposure to body fluids. Federal health officials did say, however, that the three had small breaks or other abnormalities in their skin.

Thus far, only two cases of such AIDS-virus transmission have been documented. One involved a British nurse who was infected with the virus through an arterial puncture wound, an atypical event that actually meant she received a microinjection of infected blood. The other case, involving an American health care worker, was also unusual in that the victim got a deep, intramuscular injection with a large needle visibly covered with infected blood.

Surveys of health care workers who have intense exposure to AIDS patients have been under way for several years now, and the data have been remarkably consistent in showing that those who care for AIDS patients or process their specimens show no more likelihood of getting the disease than anyone else, nor must they employ any special infection-control procedures beyond what is standard procedure for caring for any infectious patient. We can certainly extrapolate from this that anyone who has casual contact with people infected with AIDS — food handlers, schoolchildren, co-workers, and family members — is at virtually no risk at all.

Studies of the families of AIDS victims have, in fact, laid to rest the erroneous belief that casual contact is a possible risk. Family environment had been singled out as risky for the obvious reason that contact among its members is so intimate that the AIDS virus would have an easy time finding a way to infect some of them. Family members, after all, share bathtubs, showers, toilets, beds, drinking glasses, towels, razors, even toothbrushes.

But the belief that such close contact poses a special AIDS risk was quelled in February 1986 with the publication in the *New England Journal of Medicine* of the results of the largest and most authoritative study of members of the families of AIDS victims. Conducted at the Montefiore Medical Center in the Bronx, New York, the study involved 101 people — parents, children, siblings, and other relatives of 39 AIDS victims — each of whom had lived with the patient for at least three months during the time he was presumed infected.

Every one of the family members was meticulously questioned and medically examined. They were asked how many times they hugged and kissed those with AIDS, how often they shared facilities or household items likely to be soiled with body secretions. There was, it turned out, considerable evidence of intimate contact, since most of the families in the study were poor and lived in very crowded conditions. Ninety-two percent of the family members had used the same bathtub or shower as the AIDS patient; 90 percent, the same toilet; 37 percent slept in the same bed with the patient; 50 percent had shared drinking glasses; 33 percent, towels; 9 percent, razors; 7 percent, a toothbrush.

The results were unequivocal. When blood tests were taken, only 1 person out of the 101, a five-year-old girl, showed any antibodies to AIDS virus. And she, according to the doctors who conducted the study, almost certainly acquired the infection at birth because her mother had the disease. "The implications of this study are strengthened by the fact that the infection-control procedures followed by many health care workers were obviously not employed in the families studied," commented Dr. Merle A. Sande, chief of medicine at San Francisco General Hospital, in the same issue of the journal.

The duration of exposure reported was certainly sufficient, and the interactions numerous enough, to provide every opportunity for the virus to be spread within the family if such transmission was likely. Other, smaller family studies have produced results consistent with those [of this study]. Only one of 35 household members associated with 14 seropositive Danish patients with hemophilia had antibody to the AIDS virus. This person had engaged in vaginal, oral, and anal intercourse with one of the infected patients with hemophilia. The failure of the virus to spread in the secretion-rich environment of the family may in part be explained by the very low isolation rate recently reported in samples of saliva. [That study] could isolate [the AIDS virus] from only one of 83 saliva samples cultured from antibody-positive subjects, although the virus was detected in 28 of the 50 blood samples tested from the same population. The picture is therefore clear. The AIDS virus is spread sexually, by the injection of contaminated blood, and vertically from mother to fetus. Other modes of transmission are extremely rare.[4]

No one can, of course, guarantee that once out of several million times someone will not transmit the virus through some nonconventional means. Some researchers criticized the conclusions of the Montefiore study as premature, arguing that longer intervals of exposure than those observed might indeed pose some hazard, and that a much larger number of households will need to be examined to confirm the study's findings. Still, casual transmission of AIDS has not yet happened to anyone's knowledge, and the epidemic has been with us long enough to have resulted in some cases of such easy infection. There has not been even one.

Along those lines, a recent pair of bizarre cases stirred up some apprehension for a time. One, reported by the CDC, involved the first known case in which a parent caught the AIDS virus from her child, a boy who was infected through a blood transfusion. The mother, who developed antibodies to the virus but no symptoms, had frequently handled her son's blood, waste, and feeding tubes — he had been born with a severe intestinal abnormality that necessitated numerous operations and a large number of bags to collect his excretions — at home. She never wore protective gloves, and often did not even wash her hands after contact with the boy's blood and secretions. The case was, obviously, an extreme one, and the mother's contact with her son was by no means ordinary.

The other case occurred in West Germany. A three-year-old boy, infected through a blood transfusion, apparently transmitted the AIDS virus to his older brother in some unexplained way. The children's parents were divorced, and the father lived apart, so he had almost no contact with them; sexual abuse and blood transfusions were ruled out. The only possible explanation seemed to be that the younger child had bitten his brother on the arm, a bite that did not even draw blood. Though it might give one pause, the truth is that such a minor incident is a very unlikely means of transmitting the virus, and American AIDS experts were highly skeptical.

Parents afraid that their children might be exposed to the virus through bites or scratches have been apprised that there have been a number of similar incidents without any resulting infection. Microbiologist James Thomas, chief of the Bureau of Laboratories for the District of Columbia, has said that he would be concerned only if the children were engaged in some sort of direct blood-to-blood contact, such as a wrist-to-wrist, blood-brother exchange. Once again, it can be said that in virtually all cases where no risk factors are apparent, a risk factor related to some form of sexual activity or blood-product recipient becomes evident after a thorough medical and social history is taken. Casual transmission of AIDS, though theoretically possible, is never apt to pose a significant risk to the uninfected.

There is something else about the AIDS virus that speaks against its ability to spread casually: its fragility. The virus, for all its crippling capacity inside the human body, is vulnerable to all sorts of outside assaults because of unique biological properties that allow its protein envelope to be easily eaten away. It is, therefore, unlike some viruses that cause central-nervous-system diseases, which are highly resistant to inactivation by heat, chemicals, and ultraviolet light. The AIDS virus thrives in a chilly environment, and heat deactivates it easily. If a sample suspended in a fluid-filled test tube is left to stand at room temperature for twenty-four hours, it has only a 10-percent chance of surviving. While a recent new study has shown that when the virus does survive in a water-based solution of human blood cells at room temperature it can do so for up to fifteen days, it is also true that common detergents and cleansers, household bleach, alcohol, even hand soap and hot water, will deactivate it. Also, a common ingredient in spermicide, non-oxynol-9, apparently kills the virus in the test tube at concentrations 100 times weaker than those put into over-the-counter spermicidal jellies, implying that use of the spermicide might reduce the risk of contracting AIDS during sex.

This frailty of the AIDS virus outside the body can, of course, be misleading. In the case of the spermicides, for instance, they do not provide complete protection against acquiring the virus through sex with an infected person, (and neither do condoms). Also, the ability of inexpensive, readily available agents to neutralize the virus only means that the virus is vulnerable in the laboratory, or on a surface of some kind. Household cleansers have no application within the human body, where the AIDS virus depends on an intimate association with certain human cells to survive and replicate; once the virus gains entry to those cells, the unique composition of its envelope shows its insidious side.

That is why researchers who actually handle the virus — drawing it in solution from test tubes and squirting it into flasks, infecting cells with it in culture dishes, cutting it apart to extract its genetic material — take no chances with its heralded lack of transmissibility. Gingerly handling their flasks and beakers, sometimes wearing two pairs of rubber gloves and masks, they work under protective hoods that fan-filter air up and out, or in sterile, glassed-in compartments with brightly painted signs warning of BIOHAZARD or LIVE VIRUS.

But still, that is standard procedure when dealing with any lethal agent, and researchers are not usually terrified when working with the AIDS virus. "You have to recognize," Max Essex at Harvard told me, "that many people, at CDC and so on, have worked with very dangerous viruses long before this one. The idea of handling an agent like this isn't really scary in and of itself because you feel you're in control of the situation, that you can prevent infection." He elaborated:

> It's a bit like riding in a sports car. You're going rapidly, and you still feel in control. On the other hand, it's not like riding in a well-reinforced car and going slowly. . . .
> It's a bit more risky than just working, say, with *e. coli* [a common intestinal bacterium], but you feel you're in control.
> Everybody has to take risks in their lives. How afraid someone is is directly related to how familiar they are with the topic. You find people who've only worked with non-

pathogenic *e. coli,* and they'd be scared to hell just thinking about this. But you'll also find people who've worked with African hemorrhagic fever who will think this is a breeze.

In September 1987, the infection showed up in a laboratory worker who had been growing the AIDS virus in concentrations that far exceeded anything that most health workers — and certainly the general public — would ever be exposed to. An investigation revealed that faulty lab equipment and skin cuts or dermatitis on the worker's hands apparently played a role in the infection.

If there is a message in all of this, it may simply be that the human race would be gone by now if AIDS were what the general public has generally perceived it to be. The AIDS virus, for all of its bluster and all of the potency attributed to it by laypeople and some scientists alike, is far less of a threat than has been imagined. Although there is always a chance that AIDS could be passed along more easily than it now is if the virus adapts itself to its human hosts, all the evidence thus far suggests strongly that the disease will remain overwhelmingly confined to the current risk populations, and that the hard-to-spread virus is not likely to become any more contagious. (A Massachusetts General Hospital researcher told me that the chances of the virus mutating into a form that would allow it easier access to a human body were less than the chance of his suddenly becoming a star basketball player for the Boston Celtics.)

Indeed, the disease could eventually die out on its own. Already, there are signs of a slowdown. In May 1987, San Francisco's public health department noted that the increase in new infections among gay males had fallen to a rate of 1 percent a year from 12 percent to 14 percent during the peak spread period, 1980 through 1982. Such a decrease is easily explained. When AIDS first surfaced, essentially every male in the sexually active gay communities was at high risk, and the AIDS infection rate skyrocketed. Because those men are already infected, it obviously has to take longer for the virus to get into less sexually active groups, if it gets there at all.

All of this leads to the question of whether AIDS is going to spread heterosexually — which is the suggestion that always seems to be behind the ominous forecasts characterizing the disease as an impending latter-day plague. I will examine this question next, and attempt to justify my argument that there is no significant heterosexual AIDS threat — that is, no major threat of the virus's being transmitted through conventional sex between man and woman — nor is there ever likely to be any heterosexual epidemic in this country or in any other developed nation. AIDS may indeed spread *among* the sexes in the United States, but that does not necessarily mean it will do so *between* the sexes. *Some* heterosexuals will contract the disease: mostly intravenous-drug abusers, both men and women, and the offspring of those women who were pregnant when they acquired the virus; less often, the sex partners of bisexual men and of men who use IV drugs.

8

How Easily Is AIDS Transmitted between Men and Women?

CONSIDER THE FOLLOWING CASE that was reported recently in the *New England Journal of Medicine:*

A thirty-seven-year-old Cleveland businessman, married, had been making frequent trips to New York City. He was bisexual, and had had frequent liaisons with other men. In 1983, he developed signs of AIDS, but continued to have sexual relations with his wife of ten years, an apparently healthy woman of thirty-three who knew of his bisexuality. The couple had vaginal intercourse accompanied by heavy mouth kissing about twice a month. In 1983, the husband died of the pneumonia associated with AIDS, and several months afterward, the wife began having an affair with a twenty-six-year-old male neighbor.

For a year, the two had vaginal intercourse almost daily, again accompanied by intense kissing. A year and a half after her husband's death, the wife died as well — of the same AIDS-related pneumonia. Eventually, her lover, who said he was not a bisexual or a drug abuser and that he had not had any contact with prostitutes, began to show signs of AIDS-related complex. Said the two doctors who reported the case: "Although it represents only a single instance, this appears to represent a well documented example of sexual transmission [of the AIDS virus] from a man to a woman to a man through frequent but traditional sexual practices. We believe the risk of such transmission is real and that sexually active heterosexual men and women should be aware of these data."[1]

Another heralded case involved a Florida man in his seventies who contracted AIDS through blood products he received for treatment of his hemophilia; he venereally passed the infection along to his wife, also in her seventies, even though they had intercourse only once every two or three months. Still another case study suggested that the AIDS virus had been passed from female to male or from male to female several times: a Swedish seaman who contracted the disease from a female prostitute in Haiti in 1979 subsequently had sex with six other women, three of whom developed antibodies to the AIDS virus; one of the women later became his wife and she passed the infection on to their son at birth; one of the three women infected by the sailor also apparently gave the disease to her husband.

Reports such as these have, quite understandably, sent shudders through the medical community, to say nothing of the public at large. The worst fears of the AIDS doomsayers, it seemed, had come true: AIDS was no longer something that happened only to "them," but to "us" as well. And beyond the implication that anyone who engaged in casual male-female sex was now at risk, there was the larger question: Would AIDS soon begin moving far beyond the homosexual and drug-abusing communities to become, as a few scientists had been claiming, a global peril that would kill off people by the millions?

Everything in each of the aforementioned cases might have occurred just as reported, of course, if only because in the unpredictable world of sexually transmitted diseases (STDs) the potential for infection is always present, even in ways that might seem bizarre. Gonorrhea can be passed on simply by juxtaposition of the genitals without any penetration. Herpes, the only significant STD caused by a virus — most of these diseases are bacterial — can be spread from cold sores on the lips to the genitals simply by a touch of the finger. Moreover, insofar as the Cleveland case was concerned, its presentation in a respected medical journal did lend the required air of credibility.

And yes, the AIDS virus has been found in semen, and in the genital secretions of women known to be at risk for AIDS. So, since the disease is spread from one person to another through infected body fluids, it would be logical to assume that unprotected vaginal sex, which involves the exchange of those fluids, might be a route. And again, yes, prudence, even more so today than in the past, should dictate the choice of one's sexual partners, for anonymous sexual contact, heterosexual as well as homosexual, is, as they say, akin to playing Russian roulette.

Yet, the troubling cases just cited (which at this moment deserve scrutiny but perhaps, for now, no more than a place on the fairly short list of interesting, not fully unexplained, sometimes suspicious oddities that have emerged in AIDS case reporting) do not necessarily mean the roulette game is the same as when it is played with dirty, shared needles, or by a male who is the receiving partner in unprotected anal sex. AIDS is now, and is likely to be for some time, largely spread by certain well-defined forms of behavior, perhaps helped along by certain conditions and circumstances; and vaginal sex is not now, and may never be, high among them, at least not in the United States. (I will examine later why the situation may be different in Africa and Haiti.)

Fifteen people were involved in the two cases mentioned above, but only sketchy information was provided about their life-styles, or prior medical histories; few data were provided that might have implicated some predisposing factor. The Cleveland case, in addition, was presented in the form of a letter to the *New England Journal,* which means it did not have to go through the rigorous peer-review process that all the more formal reports must. In the Florida case, was age a factor? No one knows. Thus, the startling divergence of such cases in the midst of an epidemic that has had painfully precise patterns since 1981 makes it difficult to view them — at least at the moment, and unless planned CDC studies on heterosexual transmission prove otherwise — as much more than flukes, or perhaps erroneous assumptions based on flawed information.

All the evidence and well-informed speculation to date suggests strongly that heterosexuals are not, per se, members of yet another high-risk group for AIDS. Contrary to what some gay advocates, eager to take the onus off their community, are saying, the simple fact is that if a person does not belong to one of the known risk groups, he or she has very little to fear from the disease, for it is not lurking in every straight singles bar; indeed, the chance of picking up the virus in such a place is about the same as the chance of winning the jackpot in a state lottery.

None of this is meant as a criticism of the gays' sexual preference. But the fact is, many gay advocates tend to ignore that, in a sense, homosexuality and AIDS are synonymous — as are IV-drug abuse and AIDS. But, again, it is not sexual preference that draws the virus to a gay male's immune cells, any more than an addict's craving for heroin invites the infection. It is, simply, certain forms of sexual behavior engaged in by gay men that put them at risk, just as addicts' needle behavior puts them at risk. The inclination of some gay activist groups to downplay the important element of mode of sexual behavior diverts attention away from the transmission pattern of AIDS and leads to an exaggeration of the heterosexual's risk.

AIDS researchers themselves are not above such exaggeration, especially when they need money for their work. Some believe that if they emphasize that AIDS strikes primarily at homosexuals and drug mainliners, Congress and the president are apt to turn a deaf ear to their requests; on the other hand, if they portray the disease as a public menace, Washington will be more generous.

If anyone doubts that AIDS is a going business, a glance at the figures should dispel that notion. According to researchers at the University of California at San Francisco, personal medical care costs tied to the disease will rise from $630 million in 1985 to $8.5 billion in 1991. Nonpersonal costs — for research, screening, education, and general support services — will go from $319.1 million in 1985 to $2.3 billion in 1991.

Finally, with expenditures like that comes visibility, the quality that can lead to fame for scientists. Although some researchers will tell you that they have more important things than AIDS to worry about, working on a disease that has a chance of spreading to the general public and therefore gets constant media attention is in itself an enticement: one gets the impression sometimes that a few of the scientists are the laboratory counterparts of military commanders who need a conflict to keep them in the limelight while they make their reputations.

And so we have the so-called heterosexual threat of AIDS, the case histories sometimes based on rather skimpy evidence, and the scary reports, which neglect to mention that — like the frequency of breast cancer in males or cancer of the heart — AIDS transmitted via heterosexual intercourse is very, very rare in the United States and that, when it does occur, it may indeed include other predisposing factors. Four years after AIDS broke out, heterosexual men and women represented only about 1 percent of the total cases in this country.

By the end of 1986, the percentage was still relatively small: heterosexual cases were up to 4 percent of the 26,000 that had been reported by the end of that year. But in one of those skillful juggling acts that epidemiologists have been performing with the "heterosexual" category almost ever since researchers began using the African and Haitian cases as examples of where the disease might be going in the United States, the category now included foreign-born individuals with the disease — more than half of them Haitians. (In the past, the heterosexual category included only those who acknowledged having sexual contact with an AIDS-infected person or with someone in the high-risk category. Foreign-born patients who did not fit those criteria were listed simply as "none of the above.") Thus, while the percentage of heterosexual cases appeared to have risen, on paper at least, the reason was not necessarily that heterosexual transmission was actually on the rise in the United States, but because Haitians, who had originally been listed as a separate risk group (a practice abandoned in 1985 out of concern that the categorization was discriminatory and made life in the States more difficult for them), were now reclassified and boosting the "heterosexual" numbers.

The CDC made the upward revision because of what seemed to be strong evidence that the Haitian brand of AIDS was primarily transmitted by heterosexual contact. As a result, the new heterosexual category now listed 862 AIDS victims, 379 of whom were previously listed in the "heterosexual" category and 483 of whom were taken from "none of the above." Of the 483, according to Dr. Harold Jaffe, chief of the epidemiology branch of the CDC's AIDS program, all but a few were Haitians.[2]

There may be another flaw in the government's statistics. The CDC acts — as Dr. Stephen Schultz, deputy commissioner of the New York City Health Department, put it — "as simply a passive repository of data collected in a variety of ways by local health departments around the country."[3] Because it has to rely on reporting of health departments that often employ cursory interviewing techniques when dealing with AIDS patients, and thus may err in properly classifying risk, the CDC can do little more than observe that "heterosexual transmission appears likely" when someone claims he or she has not engaged in anal sex or has not shared a needle with an infected person. While the implication is left that the disease was transmitted through conventional heterosexual contact, the CDC cannot say whether the heterosexual cases it collects were actually spread through vaginal sex alone. The agency does not ask many pointed questions, and there are, therefore, very few data at the moment to correlate sexual practices with transmission.

Then there are the outright baffling cases, the ones the CDC places in the "no identified risk" category because no one had any idea how the patients got the disease. Part of the reason for the uncertainty is that many AIDS patients refuse to be interviewed, or die before the national surveillance system can get to them. However, it can be said with a good deal of certainty — again, given the steady track that AIDS has followed — that the vast majority of patients in whom no risk is identified will, in reality, have risk factors when additional information becomes available.

When CDC personnel began reviewing 1,133 AIDS cases that had initially been listed as "no identified risk," they found that there was, indeed, usually an explanation. After reviewing 591 cases, the CDC reclassified 431 of them. Of that group, 206 were homosexual or bisexual, 129 had "heterosexual contact" with AIDS victims (again, no details were available about actual sexual practices and under what conditions), and the rest turned out to be drug abusers who shared needles, belonged to other risk groups (Haitians or central-Africans), or did not really have AIDS.

It is no wonder that in late September of 1985, AIDS specialists at the CDC reported that "current modes of transmission will remain stable, and sexual transmission of the virus will account for the vast majority of the cases in the United States for many years to come. Homosexual men and persons who abuse intravenously administered drugs will remain at extraordinary risk for AIDS. The disease will probably become the major cause of death in these populations." The CDC has repeated that prediction regularly. By 1991, the agency says, 270,000 people will have been diagnosed as having AIDS. More than 70 percent will be homosexual and bisexual males, and 25 percent will be IV-drug abusers (about 8 percent of them homosexuals). Of the new cases projected for 1991, about 10 percent — some 7,000 — will be classified as "heterosexual," some of them (no one knows just how many) also drug abusers. In June of 1986, the U.S. Public Health Service could only add: "Current information is insufficient to predict the future incidence of HTLV-III/LAV in the heterosexual population."

But despite the statistical morass in which the heterosexual issue is caught, we continually read newspaper accounts — and view even more surface television "special reports" on AIDS — that do not go beyond the suspect numbers, nor beyond merely reporting what a few researchers have concluded on the basis of some very limited studies. DATA SHOWS AIDS RISK WIDENING, the *Washington Post* recently headlined a story that leaned heavily on the rise in heterosexual cases from 1 percent to 4 percent, on the African and Haitian experience with the disease, and on incredibly small studies of military families. Or consider, in the *New York Post*, DOC: IT'S SPREADING FAST, over a story about AIDS researcher William Haseltine's testimony before a senate subcommittee in which the scientist referred to an army study that found that 5 percent of the GIs in Berlin seeking treatment were infected with the AIDS virus. The soldiers, according to the report, were apparently infected by prostitutes, of whom 20 percent to 50 percent reportedly carry the virus. But nowhere in the report was it mentioned that the military is not always representative of the general population, that it is hard to get a straight answer from a serviceman, that it is advisable to say one caught AIDS from a prostitute because to admit to drug abuse or homosexuality means getting kicked out of the service.

There are undoubtedly elements of truth in all of the media accounts of AIDS cases arising through heterosexual contact, but whether these cases are as widespread and have been as efficiently acquired as some researchers claim are questions open to serious challenge. The high numbers of AIDS cases among the clearly defined risk groups, and the relatively few heterosexual cases since 1981, are two fairly good indicators of the path the AIDS virus has followed — and, probably, will continue to follow.

It must be said, though, that some scientists are not averse to suggesting that this mold will be broken. "Just wait," one Harvard researcher told me, "just give it time. It had to start somewhere, you know, and it's moving fast." When I mentioned to another virologist that anal intercourse is implicated in the majority of AIDS cases in the United States, he pounded his desk and shouted in rage, "You're not helping your country at all by focusing on that!" And when I asked an AIDS researcher at a Boston hospital whether the African "heterosexual epidemic" might be related to the widespread practice of female "circumcision" with unsterilized knives, razor blades, sharp stones, or broken glass, which can cause genital infections, disturbances in menstruation, and blood clots, he was disdainful. "Those," he said loftily, "are artificial constructs put up to reassure us falsely. The burden of proof is on those who invoke cofactors. Next question."

The key question, really, is not whether AIDS can be transmitted between men and women who engage in conventional intercourse — because, as we have seen, the theoretical potential, at least, is there. It is, rather, like the problem with nuclear reactors: there is general agreement that all of them could conceivably experience a disaster on the scale of Chernobyl, but the potential is exceedingly low. A far better, and more relevant, question is: Can AIDS be transmitted as easily through conventional sexual intercourse between men and women as it is between infected males who engage in anal sex, or via a drug addict's contaminated needle, or from an infected pregnant woman to her unborn child. Another is: Is the transmission between women and men equally efficient in both directions? These questions are important if the extent and future course of AIDS, both in the United States and throughout the world, are to be charted accurately.

While the relative efficiencies of the various sexual means of transmission have been difficult to assess because of inadequate research data, there is, on the other hand, most certainly enough epidemiological evidence to make a very strong case for a negative answer to both questions. Mainlining the AIDS virus through a contaminated needle or from an infected blood supply is still regarded as the most efficient way to get an infection. The child in the womb, exchanging blood with an infected mother for nine months, is also as vulnerable — an "immunologic sitting duck," as one pathologist characterized such a situation for me. And scores of studies have positively identified receptive anal intercourse and multiple sex partners as the primary risk factor for AIDS infection in homosexual men.

On those infrequent occasions when transmission may have occurred between men and women practicing vaginal sex, one can postulate — given the relatively few cases of such transfer, the patterns followed by other venereal diseases, and the noteworthy differences between male and female genital anatomy — that passage of the AIDS virus was probably far easier from man to woman than from woman to man, and even then occurs only under certain predisposing conditions that allow the virus freer-than-normal access to a person's bloodstream. Of the small number of cases in which AIDS patients said their only risk factor was heterosexual contact with a member of the high-risk group, the vast majority were women.

(At one point, when the CDC was listing 155 people in the heterosexual category, 137 were women and 18 were men. That, incidentally, was out of 15,000 AIDS cases reported at the time of the survey. Contact with an IV-drug abuser accounted for 73 percent of the heterosexual cases; with bisexual males, 18 percent; and with hemophiliacs and transfusion recipients, most of the remaining 9 percent. By early 1987, more than

2,000 women had been diagnosed with AIDS. The majority to date have been IV-drug users, although the frequency of cases in women infected through sexual contact seems to be increasing.)

Determining the exact degree of risk for those who practice only vaginal sex with an infected partner is, however, quite difficult, and the scant literature on the subject is full of disagreement. One estimate, by Dr. Thomas A. Peterman of the CDC, who studied 20 husbands and 50 wives who were sexually active with an infected spouse (the spouses all got the AIDS infection from tainted blood in transfusions), found that 1 of the husbands and 8 of the wives became infected. Peterman suggested that the risk of picking up the virus through a single heterosexual encounter with an infected partner was 0.1 percent for a woman and 0.05 percent for a man.[4] A more recent study estimated that a woman's chances of infection from a single episode were about one in a thousand.

The doctor who has argued most loudly that heterosexual transmission of AIDS is not only possible but easy is Major Robert Redfield of the Walter Reed Army Medical Center in Washington, a clinician-researcher who is strongly convinced that the AIDS projection curves for 1991 are serious underestimates and that no one is naturally immune from the disease. Redfield is one of the few scientists who have gathered any data to try to prove that AIDS is a bidirectional VD. He and his colleague Colonel Donald Burke were also among the first to diagnose AIDS in the military and blame some of the infections on female prostitutes.

In Redfield's view, the appearance of AIDS parallels what initially happened with syphilis in this country. "When sexually transmitted diseases occur in society, they first show up in the group that's most sexually active," he told me. "And when they get amplified to a certain point, they start to infect more and more people who are less and less sexually active. The virus doesn't care if you're a man or a woman. From its perspective, you're a primate. If you have sex with someone who's infected, male or female, you're at risk, period. This infection goes as easily from man to woman as from woman to man and from man to man."

Redfield's studies of military personnel, both male and female, are important, but too small to allow any meaningful conclusions to be drawn from them. In a spouse study, 5 of 7 women whose husbands had AIDS became infected, and 3 of them developed ARC. Although he cannot identify the means by which the virus was transmitted (blood to blood, blood to mucous membrane, or saliva to mucous membrane), Redfield says he is sure it was not rectally. In another group, he found that 15 of 41 patients with AIDS or ARC (10 men, 5 women) had apparently acquired the infection from their infected partners; again, he says, the 5 women did not have anal intercourse. He adds, moreover, that his studies of 34 married couples show that if either the husband or the wife is infected, the AIDS virus has an almost equal chance of being transmitted: 42 percent of the husbands became infected, 47 percent of the wives. (Several other more recent studies draw conclusions similar to Redfield's. Two of them, involving some 150 couples at the University of Miami and at the Montefiore Medical Center in the Bronx, found that half of the regular, longtime heterosexual partners of AIDS patients — partners who did not belong to any risk groups — became infected through vaginal intercourse; moreover, the infection apparently passed just as easily from the women to the men as from men to women.)

"One has to raise the possibility," Redfield argues, "that the efficiency of transmission may be, as with every other VD, relatively the same. Hepatitis B happens 40 percent of the time when it goes from man to woman, 30 percent from woman to man. Gonorrhea is something like 40 percent man to woman, 32 percent woman to man. So, right, the argument of the purists that all sexually transmitted diseases are more efficient from man to woman is valid. But to me, that's not significant. What the purists are talking about is the difference between 30 percent and 40 percent, and that's giving people the wrong message, and it's not enough to make any difference in your risk."

Redfield also thinks there has been far too much emphasis on AIDS as an infection related to drug abusers, and to gay men and their sexual practices.

I'm not saying the virus isn't transmitted that way. It's the assumption that that's the more efficient way that troubles me. No one knows whether female-to-male sexual transmission is more or less efficient than transmission from males to females, or among members of the same sex.

And no one really knows the efficiency of transmission by sharing drug paraphernalia. If anything, we know that needle-stick transmission with AIDS rarely occurs in health workers, and that tells me something. It tells me that you can't ignore the fact that, yes, addicts are at risk, but they can also acquire the disease because they've had sexual exposure.

I question that the use of drugs is the way that all drug addicts get infected. Male drug addicts who are infected become a major reservoir, true. And they can introduce it to females who are addicts or not. We don't know the efficiency of sharing needles, but my paper on spouses clearly shows transmission of HTLV-III is extremely efficient. Yes, the prevalence of AIDS infection has been greater in males, but we have to be careful not to interpret prevalence and efficiency of transmission as equal. They are not related. It would be remarkable indeed if HTLV-III was the first example of a unidirectional sexually transmitted disease.

But the AIDS virus — as we have seen, probably the most complex retrovirus known to man — does not necessarily behave according to the standard rules of venerealogy; and despite what Redfield calls the "negligible difference" between the 32-percent and 40-percent rates at which infected women and men spread gonorrhea, the fact remains that the gonorrhea bacterium is transmitted less efficiently from women to men. That could hold true for AIDS. It has also been argued that comparing AIDS to other venereal diseases, such as syphilis and gonorrhea, may not be appropriate if only because AIDS has not spread far beyond the risk groups. According to London venerealogist John Seale, AIDS and hepatitis B are sexually transmissible diseases only in the sense that they can be transmitted by anal intercourse. "Blood is the only vehicle for transmitting these viruses," Seale has said, "and chance abrasions of skin or mucosa are the sole portals of entry." In that respect, Seale has observed, both viruses may be similar to the common wart virus, which is spread from person to person through abrasions of the skin.

That the woman who has conventional sex with an HIV-infected man is more apt to contract the infection than he from her if the situation were reversed is rather easily (though not definitively) explained. "Think of viral load," Dr. George Galasso, a member of the NIH task force on AIDS told me. "Even during normal [vaginal] sex, the male is putting lots of cells into the female, so the possibility of infecting in that direction is greater. You can't exclude the other way, of course, because if the virus is in the female, abrasions on the penis make it possible. But the odds are that it's going to go male to female rather than the other way."

Multiplicity of partners, either heterosexual or homosexual, would, naturally, increase the risk to the woman. Many medical professionals who work with AIDS patients believe that bisexuality is an important unpublicized factor in the spread of the disease in some of those cases in which women seem to have acquired the disease from men. In a recent case in Minnesota, two women members of a sexual "swingers" club became infected with the AIDS virus after each reportedly had sex with 25 fellow club members; 2 of 5 men with whom both women had had repeated intercourse were bisexual.

There are apparently many more bisexual males in the United States than has been generally assumed, although those who pursue such a life-style regularly apparently are not numerous. But those who engage in homosexual activities a few times a year, along with their regular heterosexual contacts, or who have had sex with men in the past, represent an unanticipated factor in the risk equation for their unwary female sexual partners.

Bisexuality has also, on occasion, been suggested as a possible explanation for the high proportion of black women (52 percent) among female AIDS patients. But since fewer black men than white men admit to homosexuality or bisexuality, and given the fact that among blacks and Hispanics drug abuse is a key element in the high incidence of AIDS, the bisexuality issue may not, in the last analysis, be very significant. "Heterosexual transmission of AIDS in the United States is mostly from drug users," said a recent report in the *British Medical Journal*.

> Three-quarters of those who have contracted the disease heterosexually have done so from index cases who were intravenous drug users. Bisexual behavior is much less important. In San Francisco, where the epidemic among male homosexuals dwarfs the epidemic among intravenous drug users, three cases have been attributed to heterosexual transmission from intravenous drug users and three to bisexuality. Thus, the rapid spread of HIV in drug users appears to be the main source for any future heterosexual epidemic.[5]

(Some pathologists suggest that many cases of AIDS that turn up in the female partners of bisexual men are the result of anal intercourse — a practice that apparently is more common among women with bisexual mates.)

A woman may be more vulnerable to acquiring an AIDS infection not only because she is, in effect, a natural receptacle for large quantities of AIDS virus carried in semen, but because of some other special circumstances. If, for example, sex occurred during menstruation, the virus might invade her body through the blood; there are apparently times during the menstrual flow when the disintegrating blood vessels are open to microorganisms the same way a skin cut is. Trauma during sex — say, a bruise of the vaginal wall — may also play a role in transmission, along with any of a number of other diseases and conditions, especially those that are sexually transmitted, probably because they make access for the virus easier through lesions or by creating more potential host cells at the infection site. (Women with VD often show no symptoms, and so do not realize that they are at extra risk.)

The probability of infection can also be increased by any condition accompanied by vaginal bleeding, related or unrelated to menstruation — vaginitis, pelvic inflammatory disease, fibroid tumors, herpes, serious yeast infections, and even the stress associated with diabetes and ulcers — as well as by the use of IUDs and birth control pills, which have similar effects. (Under the influence of oral contraceptives, and during pregnancy, the cellular lining of the uterine cervix, the narrow neck of the womb, may become fragile and crumble; blood vessels, which are often opened during intercourse, provide a pathway of entry similar to that resulting from rectal intercourse.) Some post-menopausal women bleed during vaginal intercourse unless they use a lubricant; and because the walls of the vagina become more fragile as a woman ages, even those who are properly lubricated may bleed during vaginal sex. Finally, anemia, a common condition in menstruating women, indicating malnutrition, weakens the immune system, making it more susceptible to bacteria and viruses.

Generally, though, a woman's genital anatomy seems to be in her favor insofar as AIDS is concerned. Designed to withstand the trauma of intercourse as well as childbirth, the vagina has fewer blood vessels than the rectum, and is usually naturally lubricated during intercourse. Also, inside are multiple layers of platelike squamous cells that resist rupture and provide a fairly effective barrier against infective agents, presumably including the AIDS virus, which appears to require access to the bloodstream.

Some researchers argue that AIDS is also a mucous-membrane disease — that is, that the virus can be transmitted through the mucous membrane of a woman's vagina without requiring a break. A few chimpanzees have been infected by rubbing the virus into their vaginas — so-called atraumatic vaginal inoculation. Also, a few women who were artificially inseminated with donor sperm infected with the AIDS virus have become infected. But both suggestions require clarification. Insofar as the chimps are concerned, of the 50 to 75 that have gotten larger doses of the virus through conventional inoculation, not one has yet come down with AIDS. In the women's case, more data on artificial-insemination techniques are necessary before any "traumatic" event that could have sped up the infection process is ruled out.

While Redfield's studies appear to argue against any anatomical barrier ("The vagina may be rugged," he told me, "but it's not all that rugged"), and while they suggest ease of AIDS transmission between men and women, other studies have found just the opposite. In one, researchers from the departments of hematology and virology at University Hospital Dijkzigt, in Rotterdam, recently investigated 59 patients with hemophilia and other bleeding disorders requiring relatively large amounts of blood products, and 35 of their spouses, for evidence of the AIDS virus. Sixteen of the subjects, all hemophiliacs, tested positive, but none of the spouses did. The researchers selected 12 of the seropositive patients and their spouses for further study, obtaining detailed information about frequency and type of intercourse and other sexual habits from 11 of them. All had engaged in vaginal intercourse, and 5 others in oral intercourse; none used anal intercourse. Moreover, only 1 of the men had used condoms before he was informed he had tested positive, while 4 did so only after they learned they had antibodies to the AIDS virus. The researchers' conclusion: "Allowing for a three-month interval for seroconversion, it was calculated that in 10 couples, a total of 1,050–1,900 unprotected vaginal intercourses took place without transmission of [the AIDS virus]. This suggests that transmission of [the AIDS virus] from male to female via vaginal intercourse is relatively infrequent."[6]

With respect to hemophilia, which is often cited in transmission studies, it should be noted that in terms of AIDS risk for the woman, being the wife of a hemophiliac who picked up the virus through contaminated blood products may not be the same thing as being the sexual partner of an IV-drug user. For some still-unexplained reason, the virus seems to be passed along more easily via sexual intercourse if the first partner infected could blame the infection on use of a shared heroin needle.

Several studies seem to bear out the relative difficulty of contracting AIDS by having sex with an infected hemophiliac. In a recent, large French study, only about 7 percent of the spouses or sex partners of infected hemophiliacs showed any signs of infection; a CDC study found that only 1 man out of 20 husbands of women with transfusion-related AIDS tested positive for the virus, while there were only 8 positives among 50 wives of men who got the disease through transfusions. On the other hand, wives or partners of IV-drug users have an infection rate close to that of gay men who are sexual partners of AIDS victims, something on the order of three-fourths positive. Whether these variations mean that the amount of virus needed to establish an infection varies with the means of transmission, hide the possibility that IV-drug users who live with one another also share drugs, or merely indicate that more of the apparently lower-risk group will become infected over time has yet to be determined.

It is quite another matter with anal sex. The anatomy of the interior of the rectum, the lower portion of the large intestine that ends in the anus, explains to some extent why AIDS has been largely a disease that involves the common gay practice (anal intercourse is second only to oral sex in frequency among homosexuals). The rectum is lined with fragile, columnar cells that are easily damaged and invaded by infectious agents, and, like the rest of the digestive tract, it is rich in blood capillaries. Moreover, the closer to the anus, the more blood vessels there are. Thrusting an erect penis into the rectum, even after using a lubricant, can devastate the cellular layer, opening enough tears to allow easy passage of the AIDS virus in ejaculated semen to enter the bloodstream.

Although the risk to the so-called active-insertive partner in anal sex has not yet been established, it is believed to be far lower than for the receptive partner. Some clinicians believe, however, that the active partner also stands a chance of getting an AIDS infection since the opening of the penis might be invaded by infected blood from the receptive partner. Also, if the active partner has lesions on his penis, the virus might have an easier time of it.

Semen plays a key role here, and not merely as a carrier of the virus. It has been suggested that in semen, the degree to which the virus is transmitted is in part related to how many lymphocytes are there; and there are apt to be a lot of them in semen — hundreds of thousands, in fact — to attract the AIDS virus if the aggressive partner during anal sex is infected with syphilis or gonorrhea (not an uncommon situation among promiscuous gays). Says Nongnuj Tanphaichitr, director of andrology (the study of males) at Boston's Beth Israel Hospital: "When you have such infections, the production of white blood cells would be stimulated, and through some kind of leakage, they'd go out into the semen. There would be more in semen than in saliva, and they'd survive better in semen because of various nutrients — fructose, for example — that are there." Thus, another infection in an AIDS-susceptible or AIDS-exposed person increases his risk both of contracting the full-blown disease and of passing it along, especially if the receptive partner has a lot of T-4 cells clustered near the rectum.

Beyond the fact that lesions in the rectum enhance the chances of an AIDS infection, anal sex appears in a more subtle way to be an extraordinarily efficient means of spreading the disease. This is true because of the types of immune cells found in the rectum, and the variety of viruses that live in them. The colon, says gastroenterologist Donald Kotler of St. Luke's–Roosevelt Hospital in New York City, "is a filthy environment that needs constant surveillance from immune cells to keep foreign stuff out of the body." The most common cells found in the colon are B-lymphocytes, but T-lymphocytes, including T-4s, are also present. B-lymphocytes, says Kotler, are the favorite targets of the herpes family's Epstein-Barr virus (EBV), and, Kotler has found out, EBV is present in the mucosal B-cells of the rectum.

The implications for AIDS are significant, because EBV, as we have seen, is thought by some to be a cofactor in the development of many cases of AIDS, and at least one study has shown that before the AIDS virus can infect B-lymphocytes growing in the laboratory, it needs to be paired with an EBV virus. The finding might mean that a recipient's risk of contracting AIDS would be greater if cells infected with EBV were already present in his rectum. The person doing the entering would also be at risk, says Kotler, if his blood already carried the AIDS virus and his penis were to pick up the EBV-infected cells from his partner's rectum.

A further explanation of the high incidence of AIDS among people who practice anal intercourse came only in December 1986, when federal scientists discovered that the AIDS virus can, in the test tube, infect and persist in cells of the colon and rectum. The finding, by Dr. Malcolm A. Martin, chief of the NIH Laboratory of Molecular Biology, was provocative because it indicated that such cells could be infected even without any breaks in the tissue lining of the rectum that would afford the virus access to the bloodstream. Moreover, the AIDS virus was able to multiply in the cells and release additional viruses for more than ten weeks after the initial infection. That finding suggested that infected cells in the colon and rectum could be the sources of continued spread of the AIDS virus to the brain and throughout the body.

That saliva is occasionally used as a lubricant in anal intercourse also compounds a risk that does not apply to women. Now that researchers have isolated the AIDS virus in saliva (even though it may be there in trace amounts), they believe the lubricating practice might be another route of transmission of the virus during anal sex. Other practices involving the anus have also undoubtedly contributed to the AIDS outbreak among homosexuals, while sparing women. Fisting, for example, is an extremely dangerous and fairly rare homosexual activity in which first heavily greased fingers, then a fist, are inserted into the rectum; the trauma is severe, as blood vessels rupture and tiny cuts are made in the rectal lining by fingernails.

Dildos, or artificial penises, can, like fisting, prepare the way for an AIDS infection if a rectum damaged by them is then subjected to anal intercourse. Hemorrhoids, which plague many homosexuals and may be caused by the repeated insertion of an object into the anus, are blood-swollen capillaries in the lower area of the rectum; when they rupture and bleed, as they often do, the AIDS virus has a pathway in. Even the seemingly precautionary practice of douching before anal sex is dangerous, because it kills off protective bacteria in the anus. Moreover, rectal douching also greatly increases risk because it traumatizes the rectal mucosa.

While a woman may be at some risk of contracting AIDS through vaginal sex (and probably more so if some of the special circumstances mentioned above come into play), her chances of getting the disease are greater if she, too, participates in unprotected anal intercourse. Here, the anatomy is the same as in a man.

Nancy Padian, an epidemiologist in the school of public health at the University of California at Berkeley, has been studying the transmission of AIDS through vaginal and anal sex between men and women. In her most recent study on the subject, reported in August of 1987, she looked at 97 female sexual partners of 93 HIV-positive males, most of them bisexual men. Overall, 23 percent of the women were infected, a clear indication that the AIDS infection can go from high-risk men to heterosexual women. Interestingly, not only was the total number of sexual contacts with an infected partner significantly associated with infection, but so, too, was anal intercourse: female partners who engaged in that form of sex in addition to vaginal intercourse were, according to the study, 2.3 times more likely to acquire infection than were women who did not practice anal intercourse.

"The high prevalence of anal intercourse among the female partners of bisexual men," Padian reported, "accounted for much of this overall association." (Twenty-nine of the women enrolled in the study practiced anal intercourse.) "Aside from one case history, this is the first study to find an association between anal intercourse and HIV infection among heterosexuals. . . . Anal intercourse was more prevalent among women who were partners of bisexual men than among women who were partners of men from other risk groups. A possible explanation of this association is that bisexual men are more likely to engage in anal intercourse with their female partners than are men from other risk groups."[7] Estimates are that rectal intercourse is fairly common among heterosexuals, with perhaps a third of heterosexual couples practicing it at one time or another, either as a method of birth control or as a preferred sexual activity. Alex Comfort's book *The Joy of Sex* is more generous, observing, "This is something which nearly every couple tries once."

What about the male's risk if he has sex with an infected woman? Many researchers think that it is less than a woman's; they point out that few men are known to have acquired the disease that way (by early 1986, only 28 heterosexual men with AIDS seem to have been infected by contact with high-risk women), and that the gonorrhea bacterium, for example, is transmitted less efficiently from women to men than it is from men to women. Nevertheless, with the announcement in March 1986 that the AIDS virus had been discovered for the first time in the genital secretions of women ("lurks in the genital secretions" was the way one medical newsmagazine put it), attention was immediately focused on the possibility that the virus could now be spread easily from females to males.

The discovery was made almost simultaneously, by scientists at the Massachusetts General Hospital (MGH) in Boston, where the AIDS virus was first detected in semen in late 1984, and the University of California at San Francisco. (Both reports appeared in the same issue of the British journal *The Lancet.*) It came as no surprise: scientists had suspected for some time that the virus would eventually turn up in female genital fluids since it had been found in the semen, the blood, and, in small amounts, the urine, tears, and saliva of individuals exposed to the virus, who were, thus, antibody-positive.

Isolating the virus was not easy, however. For one thing, as in most body fluids other than blood and semen, the virus in female genital secretions was present only in small amounts. And, unlike semen, which is basically sterile, female secretions contain bacteria, yeast, and other organisms. The researchers were, thus, forced to add antibiotics to the samples to ensure that no foreign matter interfered with their culturing of the virus.

In the MGH study, 14 women who were antibody-positive were tested at the midpoint in their menstrual cycles (between seven and fourteen days) to protect the culture from blood contamination; the cultures were also carefully screened to be certain that no sperm were present. Seven of the women — all of whom were either intravenous-drug users or the sexual partners of IV-drug users, and many of whom were prostitutes or had been prostitutes — had the virus in their blood. Of the 7, 4 had the AIDS virus in their genital secretions. The San Francisco study, conducted in the lab of Jay Levy, involved 8 women who were either intravenous-drug users or had had sexual relations with bisexual men or with IV-drug-using men infected with AIDS. Four of the women had the AIDS virus in their vaginal secretions.

What can be made of the findings? Did they merely confirm the expectations that the virus would be found where it was or did they signal more? Could the discovery be viewed as proof that the AIDS virus is transmitted by infected women to men during sexual intercourse? Can such transmission occur during one sexual encounter, or must there be many?

The researchers were cautious in their conclusions. "We have suspected for some time that females can sexually transmit the AIDS virus," said Dr. Markus W. Vogt, a research fellow in the MGH infectious-disease unit and the principal investigator of his institution's study.

> This at least provides us with a missing link. That is, that the virus can exist in the secretions and might be transmitted. Epidemiological studies from Africa and the United States suggest that sexual spread from prostitutes to their partners may be an important way of introducing the virus into populations not now at risk. Efforts to define the risk among prostitutes are underway in various parts of the world. The public health implications of genital [AIDS-virus] carriage by high-risk women are obvious.

Said Dr. Martin S. Hirsch, whose laboratory at the MGH isolated the virus in the women's genital secretions: "Although there appears to be much less AIDS virus in the heterosexual community in the U.S. than in the male homosexual population, we believe it is too early to make any conclusions about female-to-male transmission. I believe, however, that the heterosexual community should be concerned and prudent in their choice of sexual partners."[8]

The conclusions of the San Francisco researchers were much the same. "The key issue here," said Dr. Constance Wofsy, codirector of AIDS activities at San Francisco General Hospital, "is to realize the need for safe sex if either of the partners might be infected. Our results support the notion that the virus could have infected [the 28 heterosexual males believed to have been infected by high-risk women] through normal vaginal intercourse."[9] However, Wofsy's group added that since the amount of AIDS virus found in the vaginal and cervical secretions was very low, vaginal intercourse is a very inefficient means of transmitting the disease.

The San Francisco researchers also felt that other cofactors might contribute to the spread: The virus could be passed more easily by women who have concurrent venereal infections with large amounts of inflammatory secretions in the vaginal canal. In addition, because it appears that the AIDS virus needs access to the bloodstream of the recipient, a man might contract the disease during vaginal intercourse with a high-risk woman only if he had a break in the skin on his penis or in his urethra (the thin tube leading from the bladder through the penis, and which is lined with columnar cells with numerous underlying blood vessels), through which the virus would enter the body and then the bloodstream.

One issue that keeps cropping up during arguments over whether woman-to-man transmission of AIDS is on the increase is that of prostitutes. There is no doubt that the virus is present in many of these women, and there does seem to be considerable evidence that this group may be a key factor in AIDS transmission in central Africa (nearly 60 percent of the prostitutes in Nairobi, Kenya, are believed to carry the virus) and in Haiti.

Studies in the United States have also produced some ominous statistics, indicating that 40 percent of the prostitutes in Miami test positive for the virus (AIDS infection is apparently higher in Miami prostitutes than in those elsewhere in this country), as do 20 percent in New York, and 10 percent in California. And the Food and Drug Administration, mindful that prostitutes constitute a reservoir for the AIDS virus, recently added "men and women who have engaged in prostitution since 1977 and persons who have been their heterosexual partners within six months" to the list of people considered to be risky blood donors.

But as disturbing as the link between prostitution and AIDS is, it must be considered carefully. Because prostitutes seem to be at high risk of developing an AIDS infection does not necessarily mean that they got it from infected men, as many researchers imply by their statistics; nor does it prove that they can and do readily transmit the disease to men, especially in view of the fact that the amount of virus present in the women's genital secretions is so low.

On the other hand, it has been suggested that if U.S. servicemen got AIDS from prostitutes, they got it in a sort of quasihomosexual contact — that is, not because the women were actually infected, but because they were carrying large quantities of infected semen they had received. "It's not unlikely that these prostitutes had multiple partners during a very short period of time, and performed no more than perfunctory external cleansing between customers," said one explanation that appeared in the *Journal of the American Medical Association (JAMA)*. "This would heighten the possibility that a male customer came in direct contact with the infected live sperm or seminal fluid of a prior patron, perhaps bisexual."[10]

Again, this is speculation, and no one can say just how risky having sex with a female prostitute is. One army study found that 9 men with AIDS or ARC had no known risk factors but that they had had contact with prostitutes while stationed in Germany. A number of epidemiologists have, however, questioned the respondents' reliability. A New York Health Department team found no evidence to support the possibility that some American soldiers in West Germany got the infections from prostitutes. (The same researchers had, incidentally, questioned the possibility of female-to-male AIDS spread and at the same time offered a scathing indictment in *JAMA* of Redfield's findings, calling his data "questionable," his epidemiological reasoning "unsound," and his evidence for female-to-male transmission "unconvincing.")[11]

In 1985, the team noted, nearly 2,000 registered prostitutes were tested for antibodies to the AIDS virus in several German cities. Only 17 tested positive, and half were identified as IV-drug users. The conclusion of the team: "A review of the 300 reported cases of AIDS [among U.S. troops] in West Germany indicates no female-to-male transmission within [that] country." The researchers suggested, also, that fear of being discharged from military service for homosexuality or intravenous-drug use (or both) would discourage self-reporting of such behaviors, and that the frequent reporting of contact with prostitutes may be a convenient alibi to satisfy interviewers and thus end further investigation.[12]

Redfield, who argues that his data suggest that more than 30 percent of AIDS or ARC cases among military personnel are associated with heterosexual promiscuity as the sole risk factor, replied that he was unaware of any evidence to support the oft-repeated statement that soldiers are more likely than civilians to lie to their doctors. "This statement is presumably based on the hypothesis that military patients with HTLV-III disease who admit to 'illegal activity' will be subject to punitive action. In fact, 20 percent of our patients were not on active duty and therefore not subject to military regulations. In addition, 75 percent of active-duty patients have admitted to 'illegal activities' such as homosexuality, drug abuse, and extramarital heterosexual activity, but none of them were subjected to military judicial proceedings."[13]

The last word has yet to be heard on female-to-male transmission of AIDS, but the observation of Dr. Randolph F. Wyckoff of the South Carolina Department of Health and Environmental Control bears mention here: "Overall," he wrote in *JAMA,*

> I agree that the evidence is strong to implicate occasional female-to-male spread of HTLV-III, and that for purposes of public safety, the evidence supports the encouraging of selective heterosexual activity among sexually active men and women in this country. From an epidemiologist's viewpoint, however, I feel that it is important to distinguish suggestive observations from epidemiologic proof and to recognize that more in-depth studies are needed before we can accept female-to-male contact as a risk factor for the spread of HTLV-III. This is of more than just theoretical importance in that if the spread of HTLV-III is not from females to males, but rather an associated or co-incidental activity, we may be delayed in appropriate identification and intervention should we be too quick to accept that female-to-male sexual contact is a risk factor for the spread [of AIDS].[14]

If the widespread belief that the disease goes more easily from men to women holds true, then female prostitutes may, indeed, be more victim than infector. What must also be made clear, however, is that many prostitutes are intravenous-drug users. Indeed, a recent report by the National Institute on Drug Abuse and other agencies stated that approximately 94 percent of former and active women prostitutes reported using heroin, and that more than 20,000 of the 50,000 women seeking treatment for IV-drug use each year have histories of prostitution.

Without denying that a prostitute could conceivably contract AIDS from an infected man by engaging in conventional sex, especially because she generally has multiple partners and is apt to carry some predisposing venereal infection that stimulates production of inflammatory vaginal fluids, it is a fairly good bet that if many of these women are infected with the AIDS virus, they got it from a shared needle; or, maybe, since prostitutes do not always restrict their sexual activities to conventional sex, they might have picked it up through whatever practice the customer preferred, including, perhaps, anal sex. Indeed, in one study a history of sexual contact with bisexual men was reported by 22 percent of a group of Los Angeles prostitutes, and a third of the women reported having had rectal intercourse.

In summary, then, it can be said with a fair amount of certainty that even though there is risk for men and women who have conventional sex with an AIDS-infected partner, the chances that a single such encounter will result in an infection appear to be quite low — even less so, as we have seen, for the man. On the other hand, even without in-depth studies to measure the relative efficiency of male-to-male, male-to-female, and female-to-male virus transmission, there is still a solid consensus among clinicians and researchers that anal intercourse remains the easiest way to pass AIDS along sexually. If this is true — and there is very little reason at the present time to doubt the statement — then the fears of rampant heterosexual spread of AIDS are highly exaggerated.

Redfield and others have cited blood tests of prospective military recruits to buttress the argument that AIDS is spreading relentlessly through heterosexual contact as well as through the other known methods. The numbers, once again, are disturbing. Out of 3 million tested for AIDS since the military instituted such screening, 1.6 of every 1,000 men had been exposed to the virus. For women, the rate was 0.6 per 1,000. The figures for the New York metropolitan area were more disturbing: 8 of 1,000 male applicants and 6 of 1,000 females were found to be infected. But though these numbers are 15 to 20 times higher than those for the nation, researchers remain divided about their significance.

The CDC's James Curran, who has long regarded AIDS as a bidirectional sexually transmitted disease, has been cautious about forming any broad conclusions. "We don't know how many of these recruits fall into high-risk groups," he says. "A lot of these kids are young. Some of them don't even know yet whether they're heterosexual or homosexual. They may have had a few experiences." Curran also points out that it is not unusual for those with a history of IV-drug abuse to try to join the army, and that New York City, especially, may have a large population of such young people. Thus, without knowing how many of the recruits fall into high-risk groups (and interviews with recruits who test positive and are rejected often establish that they indeed have had IV-drug or homosexual experiences), we cannot use the army's numbers as a predictor of trends in the population at large, least of all as evidence of heterosexual transmission of AIDS. (In November 1986, a New York City Health Department team reported that military recruits in the city who tested positive for the AIDS virus indeed do tend to be members of known high-risk groups.)

That AIDS is a major public health problem, thus far an incurable one, is a given. But that it is destined to break out into the general population is not. If AIDS is going to spread heterosexually in this country, its victims are likely to be those who shoot dope, both male and female, and not straight men and women who engage in conventional sex and who do not abuse drugs.

9

AIDS in Africa and Haiti

Ex Africa semper aliquid novi.

— *Pliny the Elder*

"THERE IS ALWAYS something new out of Africa." The old words apply, unfortunately, to AIDS, which has been occurring in epidemic form in central Africa since the late 1970s. That the new virus that has come to plague much of the world originated in African monkeys is generally accepted. The startling pattern of the disease on the continent, differing so markedly from that of AIDS in the United States, presented a new challenge for epidemiologists and virologists: while the U.S. ratio was about 15 men to every woman, with homosexual intercourse accounting for the vast majority of the cases here (and just about everywhere else, for that matter), in Africa equal numbers of men and women were carrying the AIDS virus — which suggested not only that heterosexual activity was behind the difference but that the pattern would eventually be mirrored wherever the disease took hold.

"To think that we're so different from the people in the Congo is a nice, comfortable position," William Haseltine told me, "but it probably isn't so. It's heterosexual promiscuity. The more lovers, the better the chance of being infected." Robert Redfield tried to convince me of much the same thing. "People say, oh that Africa, it's different. That's very colonialistic. The fact is, AIDS has moved. The infection has spread through Africa, like it's spreading through the U.S."

It is all too true, of course, that AIDS has spread with frightening rapidity throughout Africa, with an estimated annual incidence of 550 to 1,000 cases per million adults, according to recent extensive reviews of the epidemiological and clinical features of the disease on that continent. And it probably will get worse before it gets better. Because women represent such a large proportion of the cases, and because the AIDS virus can be transmitted through breast-feeding as well as through fetal blood exchange, fears have been mounting that newborn infants will represent a new and vast pool of infected individuals for generations to come.

Much of what responsible scientists like Haseltine and Redfield are saying is quite true. But only so far as the statements go. Promiscuity, both heterosexual and homosexual, does raise the risk, but as I have tried to point out, it does not do so equally among men and women in the United States, at least not so far.

But the reasons behind the spread of the disease in Africa cannot always be applied to the way AIDS is moving, or will move, in America — or, indeed, anywhere else but (perhaps) Haiti. And although, biologically speaking, we may be no different from the people in Africa, from the standpoint of sexual practices, public health, and all of the environmental and cultural factors that can promote disease, we are very different; and it is that difference that sets the African AIDS epidemic far apart from our own and makes it easier for the AIDS virus in Africa to circulate and recirculate (as "colonialistic" as that may sound). To conclude from what epidemiologists are observing in Africa that AIDS will break hugely out of its relative confinement in the United States is much too simplistic, and is not borne out by any shred of evidence whatsoever.

What, then, are we to make of AIDS in Africa? If the disease is rarely passed along through heterosexual activity in the United States and elsewhere, why is it so widespread in Africa — and in Haiti, as well — among both sexes? Answers have not come easily, in part because information is so hard to obtain. And even when it is available, it must be taken with heavy doses of salt.

For one thing, Africans have not been all that pleased by the suggestions of researchers in the West that AIDS got started in the green monkey (nor have Haitians been happy over speculation that they brought the disease from Zaire to Haiti and thence to New York through homosexual contact). Not too long ago, one Kenyan newspaper writer claimed in all seriousness that AIDS-infected foreign tourists were deliberately coming to Africa to spread the disease as part of an international conspiracy on the part of large drug companies seeking new markets for their pharmaceuticals; others have charged that AIDS is further evidence of how white supremacists try to foist their own plagues onto the hapless blacks. Moreover, on those rare occasions when African governments admit that AIDS is a problem, they are generally tight-lipped about the extent of the epidemic.

But despite the denials, the problem exists. And it is enormous. According to the World Health Organization, about 10,000 cases are now occurring every year in the AIDS belt across the continent's midsection, bringing the total to at least 50,000 since 1981, about twice the U.S. caseload so far; another 1 million to 2 million people may be carrying the virus, but are still without symptoms. And yet, actual reports from Africa itself are few and far between, and when they are made public, they give no breadth to the epidemic.

At last count (as of September 1987) AIDS cases actually reported by the Africans numbered only about 6,000 — when according to just about every other reliable estimate, the incidence of the disease in several African cities equals or exceeds that in San Francisco and New York. "The AIDS situation in Africa is something like syphilis in Europe," said pathologist Alexander Templeton of Rush–Presbyterian–St. Luke's Medical Center in Chicago. "In France, they always refer to syphilis as 'that German disease,' while the Germans refer to it as 'the French disease.' "

Cultural differences also compound the difficulties for investigators trying to assess the extent of AIDS in Africa. Many

Africans consider blunt, direct questions ill-mannered and will not respond to them. The sexual vocabulary also presents obstacles. Some translations of vasectomy, for example, raise images of castration in the African mind, and the Swahili word for plastic, elastic, or rubber, can mean a football or an inner tube, as well as a diaphragm, an IUD, or a condom. In Cameroon, native speakers use terms that distinguish among virgins, sexually-experienced-but-childless women, and mothers, whereas those who use the language imprecisely refer to all adult women as "mothers."

Adultery, in some groups, is defined very strictly: one tribe, for instance, believes that a man has committed adultery with a married woman he is not related to if he merely walks along a path with her or gives her snuff or a drink of beer; stepping or jumping over someone, or sitting in certain positions, may be treated as the equivalent of sexual intercourse or at least be viewed as an activity full of sexual overtones.[1] In the face of such cultural and language barriers, is it any wonder that the simplest questions epidemiologists in the field might ask about African sexual practices often elicit responses that are difficult to understand and to catalog appropriately, let alone draw any meaningful conclusions from?

What does seem clear is that a variety of practices and conditions may be at the root of Africa's unique AIDS epidemic — practices and conditions that do not always apply to the United States and to most other parts of the world where AIDS has erupted. Among them:

• The widespread administration of vaccines and medicines with unsterilized needles, both in hospitals and clinics and by untrained practitioners. (In poor countries, the cost of disposable needles and syringes limits their availability.) A recent *JAMA* report on AIDS in Kinshasa, the capital of Zaire (where 27 percent of the prostitutes who come to clinics for treatment carry AIDS-virus antibodies), noted that 80 percent of the patients admitted receiving medical injections before the onset of the disease; 29 percent went to traditional medical practitioners (who often inject vitamins or other nonmedicines), and 9 percent had received a blood transfusion during the three-year period before the illness. (It has been estimated that someone who receives a blood transfusion at Mulago Hospital in Uganda stands a 10-percent chance of getting infected with the AIDS virus.)

"I suspect that up to half of all AIDS cases in Africa are probably the result of needles that have been reused in health clinics, and needles used in certain tribal customs," said Frank Polk, Johns Hopkins professor of medicine. Barbara Visscher of the University of California at Los Angeles added: "You wouldn't believe how casually they reuse needles over there. You go to your local druggist to get a shot of penicillin, and the needle you get may have been used on a couple of gonorrhea victims."

• Promiscuity and prostitution. That indiscriminate sexual activity is rampant in many parts of Africa is well known. Indeed, having sex with a prostitute — most often without using a condom — is considered a status symbol. Case control studies have shown that AIDS patients have a significantly higher number of heterosexual partners than do controls, that more male AIDS patients report contact with prostitutes, and that there has been a dramatic increase of AIDS infection among prostitutes. For years, anthropologists have documented the loose state of affairs in Africa, the sexual freedom, the rituals of incestuous consummation and of pederasty, the masturbation, the active sex lives that begin in childhood. For men to have more than one wife is the general pattern; men often share wives sexually with guests or, in some of the more reserved communities, only with men belonging to the husband's age group or with a close relative; in some tribes, all of the women have experienced sexual intercourse as children, and even though adults maintain they do not approve of such behavior, they do little or nothing to prevent such sexual experimentation unless it occurs near them.

Wrote one observer of the African sexual scene:

In [some] societies, notably the Zande and the Nupe, a few men control great numbers of women, leaving many men without any legitimate mates. The only traditional societies on the whole continent for whom the ideal is monogamy are the Ethiopian Christians, the Berbers of North Africa (even though they are Muslim), the Mbugwe (a Bantu-speaking group in mainland Tanzania), and the Nigerian Daka and Jibu. For a woman to have more than one husband has been described as almost nonexistent throughout Africa. But there are instances where a woman may have several recognized mates. What is clear is that in many societies — whatever the label given by the particular society itself to the arrangement — women are allowed to have many sexual partners. This fact is a serious problem for exponents of sociobiological theories of differing male and female reproductive strategies. And this does not even consider the illegitimate affairs of women. These may be extensive, even in societies that trace descent through males, which sociobiologists believe have a lower rate of female promiscuity than those that trace descent through females. An extraordinary counter-example is that of the patrilineal Muslim Nupe, where married women are so free with their sexual favors that it has been described as bordering on prostitution.

In at least three societies, according to this authority, a widow must perform sexual intercourse ritually to remove her polluting status as a widow; the Twi of Ghana require, in fact, that before a widow remarries, she must have sex with a stranger who does not know she is a widow in order to cleanse her of the spirit of her dead husband.[2]

In such an environment, AIDS has found a firm foothold. Uganda, in eastern Africa, with a population of some 14 million and the dubious distinction of being a hotbed of infectious diseases, is a glaring case in point. There, AIDS, the disease known as "slim" by the natives because of its wasting nature, has virtually carpeted the area, and is now a true public health menace that has infected, at last count, about 10 percent of the sexually active people in the capital, Kampala.

If ever a country was ripe for an AIDS epidemic, it was Uganda. Superimposed on its liberal sexual mores, and aiding and abetting the spread of the disease that would strike it, were the problems that accompanied the nation's efforts to resurrect itself after many years of repression, violence, and civil war, brutal periods under presidents Idi Amin and Milton Obote during which women from outside tribes were raped routinely, family values and morality were eroded, and women, desperate to escape the horrendous living conditions, fled to other towns to pursue, according to one United Nations official, "lives of greater economic and sexual freedom."[3] Said one American gastroenterologist who worked at Mulago Hospital in Kampala: "There is profound promiscuity in Uganda, and a virus that takes advantage of it. The average Ugandan has sex with great frequency and with a great number of different partners."[4]

According to a recent Ministry of Health newsletter, Ugandan AIDS patients had, on average, a lifetime total of 18 sexual partners each, compared to 9 each for patients without AIDS. A journalist who visited the village of Kasensero on Lake Victoria, where Uganda's first victim of "slim" died in 1982, corroborated that assessment. When a group of natives was asked whether they had curtailed their sexual activities in light of the AIDS outbreak, the question touched off a good deal of glee. "They say they are still enjoying life," the journalist was told by his interpreter.

But the enjoyment in Africa is skin-deep. Sixty percent of the female prostitutes in Nairobi, the Kenyan capital, are estimated to be infected with the AIDS virus; in Rwanda, nearly 90 percent. Even though the disease is transmitted less efficiently from women to men in the United States and elsewhere, in Africa, because of the promiscuity — one study of men with AIDS found that 81 percent had regular contacts with prostitutes, and had an average of 32 sexual partners a year — and the accompanying venereal diseases, such as gonorrhea and chancroid, which can cause bleeding and tissue damage, AIDS may well infect African men more easily.

Indeed, a study led by the NIH's Thomas Quinn suggested a connection between AIDS susceptibility and the presence of other infections. Homosexual American males and Africans of all types were found to have higher levels of antibodies against syphilis, hepatitis B, herpes, and four other microbes than did U.S. heterosexuals. Such high levels of exposure presumably result in a "chronically activated" immune state, which might increase someone's vulnerability to AIDS.

One survey, among AIDS patients in Kinshasa, revealed that

a third reported having had at least one sexually transmitted disease during the three years preceding their illness. Occurrence of genital ulcers in men correlated with the presence of antibody to the virus, suggesting that virus in vaginal secretions may have been transmitted to a male sexual partner through breaks in the skin. Apart from contracting it directly from a prostitute, an African male may also pick up the virus indirectly. Randolph Wyckoff has suggested that association with prostitutes may predispose the male to developing another venereal disease, which requires him to seek an injection with a nonsterile needle, thus exposing him. "Compared with industrialized nations, Africa suffers inordinately from sexually transmitted diseases," researchers from the CDC and Family Health International reported in *The Lancet*.

> It has higher prevalence rates of traditional STD, such as gonorrhea and syphilis, higher proportions of antimicrobial-resistant organisms, and higher levels of complications, including pelvic inflammatory disease [PID], infertility, and adverse pregnancy outcomes. Between 20 percent and 40 percent of acute admissions to gynecology wards in Africa are related to PID. Infertility is as high as 50 percent in some areas; and as much as 80 percent of infertility is attributable to STD. Moreover, cervical cancer is the commonest neoplasm in Africa, and the most likely cause is an STD, human papillomavirus infection. Perhaps an even greater cause for alarm is the high incidence of adverse pregnancy outcomes caused by STD. Gonococcal ophthalmia neonatorum, a severe gonorrheal inflammation of the eye in newborns, is over 50 times more common in Africa than in industrialized countries. Maternal syphilis seems to cause a fetal death or a syphilitic infant in five to eight percent of all pregnancies surviving past 12 weeks in many parts of Africa.[5]

The promiscuity issue may also play a role in the Haitian AIDS outbreak. According to Warren Johnson, an epidemiologist at Cornell Medical College, the proportion of AIDS cases in Haiti that could be blamed on homosexual sex, blood transfusions, or IV-drug abuse has dropped over the last few years from 71 percent to 11 percent. His studies there suggest that the disease is now spread mainly through heterosexual contact, probably through prostitutes; one survey, in fact, found that 49 percent of 110 prostitutes were infected. Reporting on those studies at the 1986 Paris AIDS conference, Johnson said that other sexually transmitted diseases show up in about half of the Haitian cases, thus lending support to the idea that such diseases help AIDS spread.

• A higher proportion of bisexual (compared with homosexual) men in Africa than in the United States. According to Berkeley's Nancy Padian, this might explain the different African ratios of AIDS between men and women. "If every bisexual male had an equal number of male and female partners, and if the efficiency of transmission from males was the same to both males and females," she wrote recently in *JAMA,* "then the observed sex ratio of cases could be close to unity with little or no female-to-male transmission. We question whether the ratio of male-to-female cases in Africa necessarily supports the hypothesis that AIDS is primarily spread in Africa by bidirectional heterosexual transmission."[6]

The role of homosexuality and, thus, anal sex, in the African form of AIDS has generally been dismissed since it is not prevalent in central Africa, and is culturally and legally taboo in all countries in the region. Apparently, few males are exclusively homosexual and, apart from homosexual puberty rites, most homosexual behavior is among bisexual men. But there also seems to be little doubt that homosexuality is on the rise in major urban centers, both among the Western-educated middle classes and the rootless, detribalized masses who have moved in from the countryside. There have also been reports that some communities have adopted a more tolerant attitude toward homosexuality, treating it as a form of involuntary possession by spirits, thereby allowing the services of a healer to be brought to bear on the victim.

Among those who have cautioned against ruling out homosexual practices in the spread of AIDS in Africa is Frank Polk at Johns Hopkins. After he returned from a research trip to central Africa, he observed that he believed homosexuality was more common there than officials cared to admit. "It's simply far more repressed, and most often is seen as bisexuality," he said. Polk added that he felt the correct way to describe AIDS in Africa was as a heteroscxual disease, but one that is mainly unidirectional — meaning that it travels most readily between men and then to women.

• Mutilating rituals. Ritual scarification of the penis is common in some African groups (to heighten the man's sensitivity to sexual relations), as is female circumcision, a mutilating operation performed to make intercourse painful for the woman and, presumably, to help ensure her fidelity. In addition to the risk of the operation itself, each time she has intercourse she will bleed as the incision tears. Critics of the mutilation factor argue that such practices are confined to village areas, and that AIDS in Africa is primarily a disease of city dwellers. That may well be true. But most Africans living in the cities came from rural areas in search of relatives, education, or employment.

"The spread of [AIDS] among heterosexuals in Africa and homosexuals in the West may point to a common factor in their sexual practices," observed anthropologist Uli Linke of the University of California at Berkeley.

> Contact with blood during intercourse is thought to be largely responsible for the transmission of the virus among homosexuals in the United States. The same principle may apply to heterosexuals in Africa, where female circumcision is still a widespread practice. In its most extreme form, referred to as "infibulation," the operation consists of the removal of some or all of the vulval tissue, after which the two sides of the wound are sewn together, leaving only a small opening for the passage of urine and menstrual blood. Subsequent vaginal intercourse is therefore difficult if not impossible and is chronically associated with tissue damage, tears, and bleeding. Anal intercourse is a common recourse for heterosexual partners. It is noteworthy that the recent outbreaks of AIDS in Africa . . . correspond geographically to those regions in which female mutilation is still practiced. Understanding the pattern of AIDS in Africa will probably first require understanding the cross-cultural differences in sexual practices.[7]

• Malnutrition. Simon Wain-Hobson, who researches the AIDS virus at the Institut Pasteur, has said that this cofactor "is the biggest immuno-suppressive under the sun," and that poor diet among the Africans may well explain the staggering number of cases, as well as why equal numbers of men and women are being infected.[8] If it is true, as some researchers believe, that many members of risk groups in the developed countries are already immunosuppressed before they become infected with the AIDS virus, then it follows that malnourished Africans — as well as Haitians, who also suffer from widespread malnutrition — might constitute a risk group of their own.

There is little doubt about the role constant food shortages play in disease in Africa. The severity and the repercussions of the myriad diseases that plague the continent are, quite obviously, the result of a vicious cycle of unabated drought which causes famine, malnutrition, and infection. During periods of prolonged famine, communicable diseases such as typhus, measles, meningitis, relapsing fever, and diarrhea spread easily, and soon reach epidemic proportions. Such diseases, it is believed, may trigger or potentiate replication of the AIDS virus in infected people.

The peculiar nature of the diseases that are prevalent in Africa may not only promote the spread of AIDS but also explain the marked differences between the clinical manifestations of an AIDS infection there and those seen in the United States and Europe. Because malnutrition and failure to thrive are common pediatric problems in Africa, it is often difficult to distinguish AIDS-associated disease. But it is becoming clear that the AIDS virus — and perhaps variations of it that are peculiar to Africa — may be showing itself in different ways there than elsewhere. Gastrointestinal and dermatologic symptoms, for instance, are common in AIDS patients in the tropical areas, while swollen lymph nodes and pulmonary symptoms are more frequently seen in the United States. (In this country, *Pneumocystis carinii* pneumonia is the commonest infection among AIDS victims, but it is in only third place in Africa and Haiti.)

• Other cofactors. Housing throughout Africa is rudimentary, where it exists, and frequently there is little more than a straw hut in which no distinction is made between bedroom, sitting room, dining room, bathroom, or kitchen. Food is cooked in the open or in a corner of the hut, and the smoke given off is a fierce pollutant that irritates the eyes, nose, and mucous membranes every day, providing easy access for infections of the respiratory tract and the development of lung cancer.

"The spread of diseases is often made worse by overcrowding and unsanitary conditions," says Dr. Mesfin Demisse, the World Health Organization's program coordinator in Ethiopia. "These develop in particular when starving people occupy temporary shelters or build shacks on the outskirts of cities and towns. The number of people in these camps can swell to several thousand within a couple of days. If a health services system is not organized from the start or planned in advance, it does not take long for an epidemic of one of these diseases to spread very fast through the camps and take its toll in large numbers."[9]

It would seem logical to assume if that such appalling living conditions can contribute to the spread of some of the more familiar diseases in Africa, so, too, can they play a part in spreading AIDS. For even though the disease is not nearly as contagious as many others, with people living in such unsanitary, stifling proximity to one another, many of them could well be at high risk of contracting AIDS if they are carrying a disease that could increase the AIDS virus's infectivity.

Unsanitary living conditions may also contribute to the spread of AIDS in another unique way among Africans, especially among children. In July 1986, virologists from Johannesburg took note of the fact that 15 percent to 22 percent of AIDS cases there have occurred in children. (In the United States, thus far, it is around 1 percent to 2.5 percent.) The scientists pointed out that African children are continually bitten by bedbugs, and concluded, "Bedbugs would probably transmit low levels of infection, but a combination of factors could enhance the susceptibility of African children — repeated exposure to the insects, a possibly lower threshold to infection in younger children, immunosuppression due to malnutrition, and excessive activation of T-4 lymphocytes by recurrent infections."[10]

Lastly, an oddment: an explanation uniquely different from

all of those that have been put forward to explain the high incidence of AIDS among both sub-Saharan Africans and Haitians. The title of the report that offered it recently in *JAMA* bears mentioning, if only because it seems as out of place in a scientific journal as would a tabloid headline: "Night of the Living Dead II: Slow Virus Encephalopathies and AIDS: Do Necromantic Zombiists Transmit HTLV-III/LAV During Voodooistic Rituals?"

The author, Dr. William R. Greenfield, an Illinois physician, called attention to the taxonomic resemblance of the AIDS virus to the visna virus of sheep but suggested that sociological evidence might link it more strongly, clinically and epidemiologically, with the human slow-virus afflictions of kuru and Creutzfeldt-Jakob disease. Kuru, as mentioned earlier, is a fatal central-nervous-system disease seen almost exclusively in one tribe, the Fore, in New Guinea; it is spread by rites associated with cannibalism. It is also the primary cause of death among the Fore, a lethality that has been confirmed in animal experiments: chimps inoculated with brain tissue taken from human victims sicken and die with kurulike symptoms. Creutzfeldt-Jakob disease is another slow-virus affliction, also a rare one, that afflicts 1 in 1 million individuals, killing around 225 a year. Its symptoms are nearly identical to kuru and scrapie, a usually fatal virus infection of sheep — all lead to dementia, and often death.

In his book on the pharmacologic basis of zombiism, E. W. Davis of Harvard mentions a voodoo priest and his acolytes processing a relatively fresh cadaver for inclusion in a sorcerer's poison; the way they handled human brain and other tissues could easily have resulted in their inoculating themselves with infectious viral particles, which is similar to the suspected mode of transmission of kuru among the Fore. But it has also been suggested, Greenfield reported, that kuru may be transmitted among the natives in New Guinea not through eating corpses or carrion but rather through excessive and unsafe handling of infected brains.

In Creutzfeldt-Jakob disease, too, Greenfield pointed out, there is an increased incidence not only among those directly exposed to possibly infected brain tissue but also among those who have handled instruments that have been used in neurological research or surgery. "Thus might Haitians using utensils involved in necromancy, or actually employing 'powders' containing HTLV-III/LAV-contaminated remains, become infected with the disease," said Greenfield.

Even now, many Haitians are voodoo serviteurs and partake in its rituals. Some are also members of secret societies such as Bizango or 'impure' sects, called 'cabrit thomazo,' which are suspected to use human blood itself in sacrificial worship. As the HTLV-III/LAV virus is known to be stable in aqueous solution at room temperature for at least a week, lay Haitian voodooists may be unsuspectingly infected with AIDS by ingestion, inhalation, or dermal contact with contaminated ritual substances, as well as by sexual activity.[11]

In light of all of the foregoing, there would appear to be little question that AIDS in Africa does follow a different track than in the United States and Europe. Clinicians, researchers, and epidemiologists who suggest that the AIDS virus views Americans as it does the Africans and the Haitians are correct. Viruses need the machinery of cells if they are to reproduce and infect, and it makes no difference whether those cellular mechanisms are in people who live in San Francisco, in Kinshasa, or in Port-au-Prince. What is different is that the virus has an easier mark in Africa and in Haiti. To suggest that the ease with which the virus spreads in Africa or in Haiti will be replicated exactly elsewhere is to deny the mitigating factors — the special circumstances, some of them appalling — that exist in those impoverished, malnourished, disease-prone regions.

In Haiti, medical personnel and facilities have traditionally been almost nonexistent in the countryside, where the bulk of the population lives (the flight of trained medical personnel from the island nation had, in fact, reached epidemic proportions in 1968, until a government decree prohibited such emigration); in 1968, the estimated amount per capita expended for health was the lowest among 21 Latin American countries surveyed by the Pan American Health Organization.[12] Uganda spends, according to the World Bank, about $1.60 per person each year on health care, roughly the cost of a blood test for AIDS. The cost of caring for ten AIDS or ARC patients in the United States (approximately $450,000 a year) is greater than the entire budget of a large hospital in Zaire, where up to 25 percent of the pediatric and adult hospital admissions have an AIDS infection.[13]

Trying to establish a link between AIDS in Africa and Haiti and AIDS in the United States is thus not only ill-advised, but perhaps also wishful thinking on the part of some who — fearful that no one will pay attention if the disease remains associated with what the majority of people regard as an unsavory form of sex, and with equally heinous drug-abusing behavior — try to keep the disease in the forefront through overstatement. Such an approach, unfortunately, tends to hoist on their own petard those who belabor it: on the one hand, researchers and clinicians wish to reassure a terrified public that AIDS is not very contagious as diseases go — and, as we have seen, it is not — while at the same time some of them raise visions of a biological apocalypse, of a disease that can be spread as easily through one form of sex as another, and just as easily between the sexes.

As I have tried to emphasize throughout this book, the threat that AIDS poses today and for future generations is a very real one, here and abroad. But the threat is not of equal dimensions everywhere the disease has erupted, for there are important regional variations in whom the virus infects, how it does so, and why. The history of communicable diseases attests to that fact, and speaks against assuming that the wider spread of a disease can always be forecast from its local pattern. For instance, hepatitis B, which is transmitted the same way that AIDS apparently is, seems to be less infectious among Westerners than among Asians, and less infectious among Western heterosexuals than among Western homosexuals.

Though the virus that causes AIDS is found throughout the world, its mere presence does not necessarily mean we are all in grave danger of acquiring the infection, unless we engage in risky practices that practically guarantee it, or are made susceptible by adverse living conditions. While it is true that semen and blood are still the primary culprits in transmitting the AIDS virus, no matter where in the world it appears, the extent to which those two essential ingredients actually spread AIDS is dependent on behavior and environment.

"Western" AIDS, if you will, primarily strikes identical risk groups in the United States, Latin America, Europe, and Canada: homosexual men who practice anal sex, and intravenous-drug abusers who share needles. AIDS in Asia, only now beginning to emerge, has been primarily linked, at the moment at least, to imported blood and blood products, with only a few cases attributed to male and female prostitution. The epidemiological characteristics of AIDS in Africa, notably the one-to-one ratio between men and women, are, as we have seen, vastly different from what occurs in the West (and in Asia) and are dependent on conditions peculiar to Africa. Haiti's pattern seems to be somewhere between the "Western" and the "African" patterns.

As the physician-educator Sir William Osler put it, "Variability is the law of life, and as no two faces are the same, so no two bodies are alike, and no two individuals react alike and behave alike under the abnormal conditions which we know as disease."[14]

10

The Role of Cofactors

Is THE AIDS VIRUS ALONE sufficient to cause the full-blown disease, or does it need assistance? At the moment, the consensus is that, yes, infection with the virus by itself is enough, with its power to do so increasing with repeated exposures. Nonetheless, the possible role of cofactors — secondary variables that can increase the likelihood of developing the disease, that perhaps have something to do with how fast it is spread, and that, conversely, perhaps act as some defense mechanism — is under active investigation.

The constellation of specific conditions and practices that appear to be playing a supporting role in the disease in Africa and Haiti represent one group of cofactors. Others, in the form of genital ulcers and other infections in the male, and the spate of medical conditions among women, might, as we have seen, explain the relatively few cases of heterosexual transmission of AIDS that have occurred in this country. Still others may explain some of the variations between AIDS risk groups — especially why, for example, Kaposi's sarcoma has been largely a problem for homosexual men with AIDS.

A number of predisposing elements — things that work in tandem with the basic causative agent of AIDS — have been suggested, among them duration of infection, environmental agents, genetic influences, a previously compromised immune system, and coexistent infection with other viruses or bacteria. Although investigators have yet to come up with firm data to support any of these secondary causes, there is a continued keen interest in what role, if any, they may play in AIDS. Identifying that role, determining whether it takes more than the AIDS virus alone to cause the disease, would give researchers a clue not only to what conditions and practices beyond those already known increase the risk of infection, but to what proportion of infected individuals will ultimately develop the disease — questions that are still high among those about AIDS yet to be resolved. Also, if the secondary factors were known, some of them might be appropriate targets in any effort to block full-scale development of AIDS in those infected.

Number of Partners

This factor is simply statistical probability: the more sexual encounters, the greater the chance of coming in contact with an infected partner. While it is believed that a single sexual contact is sufficient to transfer the AIDS virus from one person to another, an increased number of sexual partners has been the most consistent risk factor associated with infection or the end-stage disease itself among homosexual men who are the receiving partners during anal intercourse. Studies have shown, in fact, that the proportion of infected individuals rises with episodes of receptive ejaculation — and is very high, one researcher has found, for men reporting more than a dozen partners. Another study of homosexual AIDS cases showed that those with AIDS had a lifetime number of sexual partners of 1,100, compared with 500 lifetime partners for homosexual controls, and 25 for heterosexuals.

But being sexually active is not the only issue. It would be dangerous to assume that an individual can always cut the chances of acquiring an AIDS-virus infection merely by limiting the number of sex partners. The size of the infected pool is also important; if it is large enough, only a few exposures, perhaps even one, would be enough to result in infection. As one virologist put it: "Once the pool gets more infection, you don't have to have an increase in sexual activity. You're just fishing in a well-stocked one now, and your chances of catching something the first time are very good."

Since much has yet to be learned about the cofactor of multiple exposure — and about all of the other cofactors that may move an initial AIDS infection along to AIDS — the number of sexual partners may or may not be significant.

Other Infections
A previous history of sexually transmitted diseases, which could stimulate some interaction between various organisms and the AIDS virus, create more T-4 cells for the virus to attack and reproduce in, or enable the virus to gain easier access to a person's bloodstream through genital breaks, may, as was pointed out earlier, be an important cofactor in AIDS. There is already evidence that people who have several concurrent infections, as do many gay men, may develop AIDS more easily than others. The implication is that the viruses that cause some of these other infections — such as cytomegalovirus (CMV) that is found so often in gay men, and the Epstein-Barr virus (EBV) that causes mononucleosis — might trigger a latent AIDS virus into action. Either that, or the AIDS virus first goes about weakening the immune system on its own, preparing the way for some other virus to come along and cause Kaposi's sarcoma, or perhaps another complication.

There is precedent for interaction among organisms in what goes on between hepatitis B and delta hepatitis, an unusual strain whose retrovirus was discovered less than ten years ago. Hepatitis B, with its 200 million carriers throughout the world, is far and away the most prevalent known viral infection of the bloodstream. Its annual attack rate on homosexuals has been put at between 10 percent and 15 percent. Delta hepatitis, carried by a retrovirus with a surface coating of hepatitis B, cannot function alone. It must either strike at the same time as hepatitis B or be superimposed on an underlying chronic hepatitis B infection.

For a time, delta hepatitis did not appear to be affecting many homosexuals. But the picture began to change, and it was but a matter of time before delta hepatitis began surfacing among gays in Los Angeles. What was more worrisome was what the delta strain was capable of doing when it met up with hepatitis B.

Although many gays are chronically infected with hepatitis B, their symptoms are mild, or absent. But a superimposed delta infection can lead to acceleration of the chronic liver disease hepatitis B causes, or to the so-called fulminating form, which causes massive destruction of liver cells.

That there may be an intimate association between AIDS and other diseases has intrigued scientists ever since AIDS arrived. At the Stanford Medical Center, for example, infectious-disease specialist Jack Remington has been studying a possible link with toxoplasmosis, the parasitic infection that can affect the brain and that is one of the more deadly AIDS-associated illnesses. Both the *Toxoplasma* organism and the AIDS virus are found in the same parts of the brain in AIDS patients, suggesting that they may influence one another in some cause-and-effect way. Most people infected with *Toxoplasma* never become sick because a healthy immune system keeps the parasite quiet. But somehow, AIDS ignites the invaders in up to 10 percent of AIDS patients.[1]

The possible catalytic role of another organism in AIDS emerged again with the discovery, reported in July 1986 in the *American Journal of Hygiene and Tropical Medicine,* of a previously unknown virus that appeared to be present only in AIDS patients. A large virus that seemed to bear no resemblance whatsoever to any known viruses, it was turned up by Dr. Shyh-Ching Lo of the Armed Forces Institute of Pathology in the tissues of 23 of 24 AIDS patients. But the nature of its involvement in the AIDS process, if any, has yet to be determined.

As with any find of this sort, speculation has not been lacking. It has been suggested, for instance, that the new virus could work with the AIDS virus to produce Kaposi's sarcoma. The idea is an intriguing one because the cancer is so prevalent among homosexual men with AIDS (it accounts for the initial AIDS diagnosis in a third to half of the cases) but not among other homosexual men, nor among heterosexual men, intravenous-drug abusers, or hemophiliacs with AIDS. Why such a clinical difference exists is not known, but speculation has centered on a covirus; originally, CMV and EBV were suspect, but so far, no firm link has been found. The new virus could also be behind some of the opportunistic infections that afflict AIDS victims, or it could be a harmless agent, one of those viruses that hide in our bodies and do absolutely nothing, and that just happened to appear coincidentally in the AIDS victims. It may also be a laboratory contaminant — not an unusual occurrence in tissue studies. (Investigation of the virus was continuing at this writing.)

Three months after Lo's virus surfaced, Robert Gallo's team at the National Cancer Institute announced that it had found a new virus member of the herpes family, which, because it showed up in the white blood cells of six patients, all of whom had swollen lymph nodes and abnormalities in their immune cells, and two of whom had also been infected with the AIDS virus, raised immediate speculation that it might play some role in the disease, either as a cause of AIDS or as a cofactor. The scientists named the virus HBLV, for "human B-lymphotropic virus," because it infected and killed the antibody-producing B-lymphocytes.

It is likely that the virus will eventually be implicated in some disease, since that is the case with all the known herpes viruses. But what disease, how infectious the virus is, how long it has been around, and how widely spread it is are still unanswered questions. Because three of the patients in whom it was found had lymphomas, HBLV could turn out to be another cancer virus, perhaps one associated with cancers of the immune system, such as lymphoma and Hodgkin's disease. There have also been suggestions that the new virus may attack the central nervous system, or, like EBV, cause a short-term mononucleosis.

HBLV's link, if any, to AIDS is, at this stage anyway, also hazy. Just because it has been found in AIDS patients does not mean it is associated with the disease, any more than Lo's virus can be linked to AIDS by its mere presence in those with AIDS. Gallo himself emphasized that there was no evidence that HBLV causes AIDS, or is even a cofactor, adding that all AIDS patients do not have it in their systems. "Clearly," he concluded after his team's report was made public, "you can get AIDS without it."[2] Nonetheless, Gallo planned to study its effect on patients already infected with the AIDS virus to determine if it might speed up progress of the disease, or make it more severe.

Another of Gallo's viruses, his earlier HTLV-I, also turned up in a sixty-five-year-old black man with a ten-year history of bisexual activity who had all the clinical signs of AIDS-related complex. What such a concomitant infection means is still unclear, and researchers are not certain whether patients with both infections have symptoms characteristic of the two viruses, or have a totally different clinical picture. "Although dual infection may not be very common," Gallo's team reported,

> the fact that it can occur may be an ominous sign of future complications of HTLV-III-related disease. Although HTLV-I is endemic in only certain parts of the world and in the United States is present — for the most part — in only a small percentage of American blacks, the appearance of HTLV-III infection in such populations may lead to new forms of neoplastic transformation and complications not previously appreciated. It is very possible that HTLV-III may accelerate lymphoid neoplasia induced by HTLV-I or HTLV-III. An awareness of these complications in areas where HTLV-I is endemic is necessary as the HTLV-III epidemic spreads.[3]

(In May 1987, NCI scientists found a strikingly high incidence of HTLV-I in drug abusers in New Orleans and New Jersey, indicating that the virus, like the AIDS virus, can be spread on shared needles.)

Another virus, one that causes African swine fever, a devastating livestock disease, has also been under investigation as a possible cofactor in AIDS. It came under suspicion in 1986 after biochemist John Beldekas, then at Boston University, and Jane Teas of the Human Ecology Association, reported a link between the two diseases, noting that symptoms of human AIDS patients closely resembled those of pigs infected with the swine fever virus. Moreover, Beldekas turned up evidence of swine fever infection in serum drawn from both pigs and some AIDS patients in Belle Glade, Florida, an impoverished town forty miles from Palm Beach that has gained some notoriety as the unofficial AIDS capital of the world. Though it has a population of only 20,000, Belle Glade had recorded 80 cases of AIDS by October of 1986, a per capita incidence comparable to that of San Francisco and New York City.

Beldekas's findings, coupled with the results of a New York City Health Department test of healthy blood donors revealing that 4.5 percent of the samples had antibodies to the swine fever virus — an indication that there could have been exposure to the disease — drew the attention of the CDC and the U.S. Department of Agriculture. (Beldekas had also suggested that the AIDS virus might infect pigs.) Subsequent investigations by both agencies found no evidence of African swine fever in the suspect herd of pigs, nor in a group of patients who either had AIDS or had been infected with the AIDS virus but showed no symptoms. The researchers also could not find any AIDS virus in the pigs. Beldekas's reaction was that he believed the CDC testing methods differed from his, and that the results may not have been comparable. "I am not wedded to this theory," he said, "but I want to see it properly tested."[4]

Immunosuppression
Early on, it was proposed that because the mysterious new disease was showing up primarily among male homosexuals, it could be explained by examining all of the practices common to that group, especially ones that might weaken their immune systems, predisposing them to the disease. Essentially, this view meant that AIDS was itself an opportunistic infection, one that was occurring only in victims who were already immuno-compromised by such agents as hepatitis B and cytomegalovirus, by repeated exposure to enormous quantities of sperm (which has the ability to inhibit immunologic killing power), or by some inherited metabolic deficiency.

"Homosexual men, intravenous drug abusers, haemophiliacs, and newborn children (particularly with incompatible blood groups) all have one characteristic in common — they may be chronically immunosuppressed by antigen overload, multiple infections, drugs, or, in the case of infants, [they are] immuno-naive," Jay Levy and John Ziegler of the University of California School of Medicine in San Francisco reported in *The Lancet* in 1983.

> Over the past 10 to 20 years, the gay community has engaged increasingly in social practices that encourage multiple sexual contacts and use of drugs. These activities are reflected in a rising incidence of sexually transmitted diseases, particularly from parasites and viruses. These factors, as well as others . . . can be profoundly immunosuppressive and predispose to severe secondary infections — for example, by the postulated AIDS agent. Likewise, intravenous drug abusers have abnormal T-cell ratios and are prone to multiple infections, particularly viral illnesses spread by contaminated food. Further, an altered immune status has been observed among haemophiliacs who are heavily transfused with blood products. Finally, the immune system does not become mature until the sixth to twelfth month of life. This theory predicts that AIDS will eventually be encountered in other exposed immunodeficient individuals, including the chronically ill or elderly with lymphopenia (particularly those with T-cell abnormalities), patients with autoimmune disease or cancer, and those receiving organ transplants after administration of immunosuppressive drugs. . . . Conversely, this hypothesis would predict that many healthy people have already been exposed to this new agent, either through transfusions or through direct contact with other infected individuals. Because they have a normally functioning system, they do not get AIDS.[5]

It was a logical explanation, and one that still crops up when the question is raised about why AIDS still does not erupt in the majority of the individuals infected. Certainly, if the co-factors that are at work in Africa and Haiti — the poverty, the malnourishment, the prior diseases, the generally poor standards of health — are valid, as many believe them to be, then any AIDS infection may well have an easier time getting started and progressing to the ultimately fatal disease in individuals who are, in effect, already ill because their immune systems are down.

One interesting suggestion about the role of a depressed immune system in AIDS was offered in the spring of 1986 by a team of Japanese researchers studying a hormonelike substance, prostaglandin E2 (PGE2), which is found in virtually all body tissues, but in especially large quantities in human semen. After corroborating, from previous scientific reports, that PGE2 acted as an immunusuppressor, the Japanese scientists concluded that the reason semen contains so much of it is to prevent sperm from being rejected by the uterus; such rejection would, of course, prevent fertilization. In the uterus and vagina, the researchers suggested, PGE2 is retained; but in the rectum, it is easily absorbed into the blood.

The conclusion of the team leader, Dr. Osamu Hayaishi of Osaka Medical College, was that the large amount of PGE2 absorbed through the rectum during anal sex could lead to immunosuppression in homosexual males, thereby increasing their risk of contracting AIDS. The hypothesis, which has been tested only in male and female rats and must still be confirmed in humans, may explain not only why male homosexuals are so vulnerable to AIDS, but why women — whose immunity is, according to Hayaishi, originally superior to that of males because of genetic and hormonal regulation — appear to be less vulnerable when they are exposed to the virus through vaginal sex.[6]

Another link between changes in the immune system, a cofactor (psychological stress), and the recurrence of disease (in this case, genital herpes) was established in 1985 at the University of California at San Francisco, where health psychologist Margaret Kemeny evaluated 40 persons with genital herpes over a six-month period. She analyzed several variables, including measures of stressful life events (daily hassles, anticipated stress), life goals, coping measures, social support, and changing health habits. Blood samples were drawn from the subjects each month so that the investigators could look at possible stress-induced immunological changes.

According to the preliminary findings, subjects with the highest levels of stress suffered the highest rates of herpes recurrence and had changes in their immune systems, notably in the number of helper T-cells in their blood. Moreover, the recurrences were most likely to occur in the month following a major stressful event — such as the death of a family member, losing a job, failing an exam, or moving — or in the month following the anticipation of a stressful event.

"Based on our preliminary data," Kemeny reported,

> we can conclude that stress and psychosocial processes are strongly correlated with T-cell subpopulation numbers in our subjects with herpes, and the level of stressful life experience and anticipated stress can predict when a person will have a herpes recurrence. It is interesting that different psychosocial processes are related to different components of the immune system. This is very important, and points to the necessity for measuring more than one aspect of the immune system, preferably many, in stress studies. This differential relationship to the immune system has fascinating implications. It may be that both helper and suppressor T-cell numbers must be altered in order to create an environment conducive to certain diseases or their progression. If so, and if one T-cell subpopulation is to some extent affected by stress, and the other is affected by social support, then alterations in social support may be required in order for stress to increase physiological vulnerability. On the other hand, alterations in stress level may be required before social support can have any influence on physiology.[7]

There may well be implications here for AIDS. There is no doubt that living with even the threat of the disease hanging over one's head — a threat that may stem from having had a sexual encounter with someone infected with the virus, from sharing a heroin needle, or from being informed that the blood received in a transfusion was tainted — can be psychologically devastating. Even without symptoms, the very possibility that the virus may have entered one's system is enough to paralyze a person with fear. If there is, indeed, as the researchers have shown, a direct association between stress and immune function, the intensity of that stress might very well determine whether someone who has had a questionable contact will develop AIDS or one of the diseases associated with it.

On the other hand, as noted earlier, the consensus is that infection with the virus alone is enough to cause AIDS — that it is the virus that severely damages the immune system, whether the system was previously impaired or not. There is, of course, strong evidence in support of this view. For instance, although there was clinical and laboratory proof of cellular immune dysfunction in each of the cases of AIDS that were turning up in homosexual men, investigators were learning that not all of the victims had a history of underlying immunosuppressive disease or therapy.

Then there was the curious connection between the nitrites amyl and isobutyl and immune-system breakdown. These recreational drugs, sold on the street in vials and known as poppers, were widely used by gays who sniffed them in the belief that they increased the intensity of an orgasm. Some researchers had found that inhaling these substances impaired the immune system and, thus, may have played some part in the development of Kaposi's sarcoma. But not all of the AIDS victims had used poppers, and other studies were finding no relationship between the substances and AIDS whatsoever. There were, however, indications that those who did use the alleged aphrodisiacs also had many sex partners, a practice that, of course, put them in grave danger of contracting disease. Nitrites were a factor, it seemed, but only an indirect one in that they, like the use of alcohol, heroin, and marijuana, might have impaired good judgment.

It was the appearance of the hemophiliac AIDS cases, among other things, that seemed to dismantle such theories as immune-overload and poppers, and thus provided what appeared to be the answer to what had become a conundrum like "Which came first, the chicken or the egg?" Investigators began leaning toward the idea that this new risk group, the hemophiliacs, was most likely being exposed through something in the blood products they were using, and that this agent was causing AIDS in them, and doing so uninfluenced by any previous immune dysfunction or other predisposing factors. The notion of a single, transmissible, infectious agent that was not associated only with something damaging to gays — poppers, previous infections, weakened immune systems — began to take hold. (Others have suggested, however, that hemophiliacs are already sick individuals, that their illnesses may have caused, or been caused by, immune damage, or that repeated exposure to transfused blood products may have been the cause of such damage. Lending some credence to this view is the fact that immunologic defects, including lower natural killer-cell function, have turned up in nonhemophiliac adults who received multiple blood transfusions.)

Also, evidence was mounting that an AIDS-virus infection required some kind of immunostimulation, rather than a suppressed immune system in the host, in order for the virus to become activated and thus be able to grow in the host and spread through its cellular population. Such stimulation might be provided by repeated infection with the virus, perhaps through virus-rich semen, or transfusions. But researchers still do not know just how many virus particles are necessary to start up an infection, just as they do not know what cofactors, if any, act in conjunction with the AIDS virus to determine whether it merely infects and allows its host to remain symptomless (for a time or — more unlikely, given the current pattern of the disease — for life) or whether it kills him.

And there the issue remains for the moment. But it should be noted that although the cellular side of the science of immunology goes back to the Russian-born biologist Elie Metchnikoff (1845–1916), who gave us the terms *phagocytes* and *phagocytosis,* the immune system remains an incredibly complex network of cells and interactions that is still poorly understood. Its role as a cofactor in AIDS is also still unclear. But, unquestionably, there is one. The meshing of the immune system and our ability to function, physically and mentally, has been too well established to neglect its importance in a disease such as AIDS, which not only ruins those natural defenses but may also take advantage of them when they are in a weakened state. The fact remains that whatever it is that influences AIDS-virus activity is unknown.

What is clear, though, is that the virus can leap easily from a resting state to one of intense activity, resulting in disease manifestations of varying severity. Thus, while doing so may never prevent AIDS, or cure someone who has it, it is still imperative that individuals who are fearful of contracting the disease because of their contacts, or who have had a questionable contact over the past few years, pay attention to maintaining as high a level of health as possible, seeing to it that they do not become malnourished, are prudent in the use of alcohol, avoid all the drugs that have been linked, even superficially, to AIDS, get adequate amounts of sleep and exercise, and try, at least, to reduce stress levels. Such an approach may well prove to be as important in fending off an AIDS infection as avoiding unsafe sexual practices and shared needles.

Duration of Infection

It would be most uplifting if researchers could tell those infected with the AIDS virus that after a certain time has lapsed, their chances of developing the disease itself will decrease. This, unfortunately, is not the case. In fact, the exact opposite may be true. As time passes, it appears, the risk increases substantially. AIDS cannot be waited out, like the flu. Although disease experts have no way of knowing just what percentage of people who have been infected will develop AIDS over, say, fifteen or twenty years, they are predicting that between 20 percent and 50 percent of those infected will go on to contract the disease within five to ten years of infection.

In a recent three-year study of 726 homosexuals from the Vancouver, British Columbia, area, a notable difference between AIDS patients and a control group without symptoms that tested positive to the virus was earlier sexual contact in the endemic areas of New York, San Francisco, and Los Angeles. "Seropositives with 20 or more sex partners in those areas in the five years prior to enrollment were almost three times as likely to develop AIDS as were those with fewer than 20," said Dr. Martin T. Schechter, an assistant professor of health care and epidemiology at the University of British Columbia. "We think that means that people with a lot of earlier sexual contacts have been infected longer and that earlier infection is probably one of the most important risk factors in determining who will develop AIDS in a given period."[8]

Age

Because the predominant mode of transmission is sexual, 90 percent of all AIDS victims throughout the world are between the ages of twenty and forty-nine; 50 percent are between thirty and thirty-nine. In New York City and San Francisco, AIDS has emerged as the most important cause of premature death among single males twenty-five to forty-four years old. Most IV-drug users, the second-largest risk group, are also young.

But does a person's age have any direct relationship to AIDS? A new study by California researchers suggests that it does, and for several reasons. As of September 1986, older infected men living in the San Francisco area appeared to be four times as likely as younger infected men to have progressed to full-blown AIDS: only 5 percent of infected men between the ages of twenty-nine and thirty-nine had developed the disease, but 20 percent of those thirty-five to forty-four had done so. The scientists, who reported their findings at an AIDS conference in Washington, D.C., in June of 1987, suspect that age at the time of infection may partly determine how well an individual's immune system can stem the progression of the disease; but they found that other factors may also be at work. For instance, men aged thirty-five to forty-four were, in general, more apt to have used poppers; they also tended to have a more extensive history of certain sexually transmitted diseases, specifically gonorrhea, syphilis, and amebiasis (amebic dysentery).[9]

Age puts some other individuals more at risk. They are the very young, especially those in utero, whose numbers are sure to swell as more women acquire an AIDS infection; when these women become pregnant, they can easily pass the virus along to their children through blood leaking through the placenta. No one yet knows what the chances are of an infected mother transmitting the AIDS virus to her offspring, but in Africa, where 15 percent of the women are estimated to be infected, it has been suggested that the children of infected mothers have a 50-percent chance of being born with the infection.

A child might also pick up the virus shortly after birth, if he or she is breast-fed by an infected mother (thus far, there has been but one such report) or receives a contaminated blood transfusion. Transfusion-associated cases among infants are less common nowadays thanks to blood screening, but newborns, especially the premature, are more apt to require a blood transfusion than older children. One study found that three times as many red-cell transfusions were, in fact, required per day in newborns, and another that 25 percent of 4,906 infants received transfusions, more than two-thirds of them multiple transfusions; yet another, in a large pediatric hospital, found that 33.5 percent of 3,056 transfusions were given to the newborn.

"[Speculation] about susceptibility of infants and children is that the amount of [virally contaminated blood] administered relative to the infant's total blood volume may result in a single large transfusion from a single donor," says Dr. Naomi L. C. Luban, chief hematologist at the Children's Hospital National Medical Center in Washington, D.C.

> Multiple aliquots [exact portions] of blood from a single infected donor during the course of the accepted shelf life of a transfer pack or unit of cells may be administered to a single infant and this may be the equivalent of a single exchange transfusion. Evaluation of cluster cases where infants have received small amounts from a single infected donor may assist in adequately answering this hypothesis, or provide new insights, although data to date would indicate that tiny amounts of transfused blood are capable of transmitting HTLV-III virus.[10]

Thus far, some 350 children under age thirteen, comprising approximately 1.5 percent of all U.S. cases, have become statistics in the nation's AIDS epidemic; half are children under one year old, and 61 have died; another 1,000 may be infected without showing any symptoms. According to the National Academy of Sciences' Institute of Medicine, of all the pediatric cases, approximately 54 percent have been the children of IV-drug abusers, an additional 10 percent are children of parents who have AIDS or who are in AIDS risk groups, 15 percent received blood transfusions, 4 percent had hemophilia, and 13 percent have Haitian-born parents.

"Infants who acquire their infection from an infected mother are generally the offspring of female IV drug users, female sexual contacts of male IV drug users, female sexual partners of bisexual males, and women from Haiti or Central Africa," the academy reported in 1986.

As [AIDS infection] continues to spread within the general heterosexual population, it would be expected that more [infected children] will be born to women with multiple sexual partners or to women whose male sexual partners have had contact with multiple sexual partners. Thus, pediatric AIDS may serve as an important marker of the heterosexual spread of [AIDS] infection. In addition, it is theoretically possible that some [infected children] may survive to sexually active adulthood, thereby constituting a continuing reservoir of potential infection.[11]

AIDS in children follows a different pattern than it does in adults. Kaposi's sarcoma, for instance, is rare among this group, but the children seem to be more prone to severe forms of various bacterial infections, such as staph, strep, and meningitis, than to the opportunistic infections seen among adults; 50 percent to 80 percent may develop central-nervous-system abnormalities; others have facial and cranial defects (abnormally small heads, prominent foreheads, and flattened nasal bridges), and still others suffer from calcification of their brain tissue, a condition found also in older children with Down's syndrome. AIDS children may also be developmentally impaired, unable to stand, sit up, roll over, even utter single words, at the usual predictable times. Sometimes, AIDS-infected children go downhill rapidly. Other times, they appear to do fairly well for several months to a year, then develop a slow form of brain disease and get progressively and slowly worse.

Anita Belman of the State University of New York in Stony Brook has described one child who could stand with assistance when she was a year old. By sixteen months, she had developed a lung infection of the sort that usually accompanies AIDS, and for the next eight months she was not able to acquire any additional language or cognitive skills. At age two, she developed another infection, a treatable one, but then regressed to the developmental level of a seven- or eight-month-old infant. "I think," says Belman, "that the immature nervous system may be more susceptible to injury, whether it be the AIDS virus or metabolic derangements. Some children have a wasting syndrome, even when you are giving them parenteral [from outside the intestine] nutrition. They have signs of losing fat and protein, and, in a developing nervous system, this may play a very big role."[12]

Not only a developing nervous system, but an immature immune system with poor antibody response and lowered T-cell response to antigens is a characteristic of newborns; this may explain the special vulnerability of infants, more so the premature baby, to AIDS-virus infection. If that is so, then the argument in favor of a weak immune system that predates an AIDS infection, and indeed influences the progress of the disease, may be an important factor in the very young, one that might not apply in adults. Says Naomi Luban: "Repeated antigenic stimuli by infusion of blood and blood products, hyperalimentation solutions containing lipids and protein [given for nutritional reasons], intercurrent bacterial or viral disease, or both, and other unknown antigens may result in immobilization of host phagocytic defense and easy acquisition of HTLV-III, a theory not yet confirmed."[13]

Race
It seems unlikely, given the scope of the AIDS epidemic, that any one racial group is more susceptible than another — at least not as a direct result of membership in a particular race (again, any more than being a homosexual per se means that someone so inclined has been singled out). Some diseases do, of course, afflict certain races. But these are genetic disorders, such as Tay-Sachs disease, the nervous-system disorder that occurs chiefly among Jewish children; thalassemia, a form of anemia that occurs in children of Mediterranean parents; and sickle-cell anemia, which primarily affects blacks. The AIDS virus, like all other viruses, is color-blind, and its ability to infect is not based

on any genetic predisposition of its host, but on finding a living cell in an appropriate species in which it can reproduce. The species it prefers is human.

Nonetheless, a racial element has been injected into the AIDS crisis. It stems from the fact that blacks and Hispanics account for around 40 percent of the AIDS cases in the United States (25 percent black, 14 percent Hispanic), a disparity made sharper when one considers that the two groups together comprise only 18 percent of the population. Around 60 percent of the 350 children with AIDS are black, 30 percent are Hispanic. In New York City, 94 percent of pediatric AIDS patients are black or Hispanic. As of February 1986, half of the women with AIDS were black, and 25 percent were Hispanic; blacks who volunteer for military service are infected with the AIDS virus at four times the rate of white military recruits.

What do the numbers, which reflect on a minority of the U.S. population, mean? No rational individual could suggest that being black or Hispanic is a direct cofactor in the development of AIDS, any more than he or she could argue that red-haired individuals are at greater risk of becoming infected with gonorrhea because of the color of their hair. What then?

For a time, when the media first began to notice the disproportion in the AIDS numbers, the answer leaned toward waffling, and the subject was apt to be handled with kid gloves. "We're still analyzing the data," said a spokesman at the Walter Reed Army Institute of Research, when the army was first seeing more evidence of AIDS virus in black volunteers than in whites. "We're not at the bottom of this yet."[14] "No matter what you do," said another source, "someone is going to charge racism. If you don't report the information, someone is going to say it's for racial reasons. If you do report it, someone else will say the same thing."[15] Others suggested that blacks generally suffered more from infectious diseases than do whites, or simply that blacks and Hispanics were more prone to AIDS because they lived in major urban areas, where AIDS was most prevalent.

Eventually, the reason behind the variance was made clear. Drugs were the big factor — a circumstance not difficult to understand considering that, according to the National Institute on Drug Abuse, some 70 percent of the nation's 1.28 million IV-drug addicts are black or Hispanic. Of the nation's whites who had AIDS, about 85 percent were gay, and only 8 percent were drug abusers. But among black AIDS victims, harder hit than the Hispanics, it was another story. More than 42 percent abused IV drugs. "In minority populations," said Dr. Harold Jaffe, chief of the CDC's AIDS epidemiology program, "AIDS is a disease particularly affecting male and female intravenous drug users, their sexual partners, and their children. This issue has been largely unappreciated. The stereotype of AIDS is that it's a disease of middle-class white men. That has prevented people from seeing it as also a minority health problem."[16]

No one is more aware of that than Dr. Alyce Gullattee, director of Howard University Hospital's Institute for Drug Abuse and Addiction, who tells her drug patients that they are setting themselves up for an early death. IV-drug abusers, she says, may pose a greater risk of spreading the virus to the general public than homosexuals since they touch so many lives and generally have children more frequently than homosexuals or bisexuals. Because they can be heterosexual, homosexual, bisexual, or prostitutes — a "microcosm of the population," as Gullattee puts it — the IV-drug abusers may indeed pose a greater risk of spreading the AIDS virus to the general public than homosexuals.[17]

Insects

From time to time, reports have implicated a variety of insects — mosquitoes, cockroaches, ticks, and tsetse flies — in the transmission of AIDS (bedbugs were mentioned earlier). Most of the reports emanate from Africa and from the Florida town of Belle Glade. Thus far, however, there are not enough data to confirm that insects can transmit AIDS, nor to assign insects a role as a cofactor in the disease. Still, the reports are intriguing, and could have important immunological implications.

Mark Whiteside of the Institute of Tropical Medicine in North Miami believes that the high incidence of AIDS in Belle Glade (and in central Africa, for that matter) cannot be explained unless environmental cofactors, especially mosquito infection, are considered. Whiteside says: "I don't buy the arguments that AIDS is caused by one virus that travels solely through the blood or by sexual contact. Every major epidemic in history has been linked to environmental factors."

The rationale for that view stemmed from early indications that a large number of the AIDS cases in Belle Glade did not seem to fit the model of how the disease is ordinarily spread: while a number of the cases belonged to one of several high-risk groups, many others did not seem to fall into any high-risk category. On the surface, at least, it appeared that the pattern of AIDS in Belle Glade was unlike that elsewhere in the United States; if that were so, it could have grave implications for non-drug-using heterosexuals.

But proposing that mosquitoes transmit the disease is quite different from actually proving it. When the CDC examined serum samples taken from residents of Belle Glade's poor neighborhoods, they could find no relationship between AIDS infection and infection with arboviruses, viruses transmitted by certain kinds of mosquitoes. If there had been a correlation, antibodies to the arboviruses would have turned up.

Few AIDS researchers accept Whiteside's theory, mainly because it presumes either that the AIDS virus can replicate in mosquitoes as do other organisms, like the parasite that causes malaria, or that a mosquito can pick up AIDS-contaminated blood by biting an infected person and transfer it to a healthy person by biting him. Both hypotheses, at this point, seem unfounded. "We know the AIDS virus is unusually picky in the kinds of cells it chooses to live in," said the CDC's Jaffe, "so it's unlikely that it could live in insect cells, which are very different from human cells in morphology and function." Jaffe was also skeptical of the notion that a mosquito could be a carrier. "Health care personnel who've been stuck with a contaminated needle," he said, "generally get more blood than a mosquito could transmit." And they almost never get AIDS. Moreover, even if a mosquito could pick up AIDS virus on its mouthpart, the virus, given its fragility, would die within a short time. (One recent study conducted in collaboration with the

National Cancer Institute found that although mosquitoes retain the AIDS virus in their systems for two or three days after an infected-blood meal, there was no evidence that the virus could multiply inside the insects or that the insects were able to transmit the virus.)

Thomas Quinn of the National Institute of Allergy and Infectious Diseases has also taken a dim view of the role that insects might play in transmitting AIDS. "There is no direct evidence yet for arthropod transmission of [the AIDS virus] in Africa, nor in the United States, where infection occurs in some areas of substantial arthropod densities," he noted in his report on AIDS in Africa.

> Malaria, a vector-borne disease, is particularly common in children between one and 24 months old in Kinshasa, but among 44 [AIDS-virus-positive] children in this city, 43 [98 percent] had other, known, risk factors for AIDS, including birth to an [AIDS-seropositive] mother, a history of blood transfusion, and frequent exposure to unsterilized needles. In addition, the lack of evidence for increased exposure to [the AIDS virus] among nonspousal household contacts of AIDS cases suggests that insect transmission does not occur over short distances (for example, by bedbugs, lice, or mosquitoes with interrupted feeding). Because of the low titer of [AIDS virus] in the blood of infected persons and the small amount of blood ingested by an insect, mechanical transmission of [AIDS] by insect vectors seems unlikely, particularly in view of the fact that hepatitis B, which is more readily parenterally transmitted, has not been found to be transmitted by arthropods.[18]

One cannot positively rule out the potential for AIDS-virus infection through a bloodsucking insect, particularly when a noninfected person lives in extremely close quarters with an infected person and there are enormous numbers of mosquitoes. In some parts of Africa, for example, a person might be bitten 200 to 300 times in one night; the chances that a mosquito might acquire infected blood are thus improved.

"Repeated exposures to certain insect-borne viruses are one of the things that lead to a weakening of the body's defenses over time," Whiteside says. "When the cellular immune apparatus is broken beyond repair, certain opportunistic infections and cancers come along which are collectively called AIDS." AIDS, he emphasizes, results from the interaction of more than one viral agent, adding that previous research has shown that insect-borne viruses can activate retroviruses in animals. Moreover, he maintains, studies have also demonstrated that animal retroviruses, such as bovine leukemia and equine infectious anemia, are transmitted mechanically to other animals by insects in conditions of crowding and in areas with an abundance of insects.[19]

But as provocative as the mosquito theory is, it would appear, at this stage of the AIDS outbreak, that closer examination of some of the baffling cases that raised suspicions of insect-borne infection may reveal them to have been caused by the risk factors that are the source of virtually all AIDS infections. In fact, that seems to be the case in Belle Glade. In July 1987, the CDC announced that its studies had turned up no evidence that AIDS cases had been caused by mosquitoes, and that even in areas where the insects abound, the virus does not infect children, who would most certainly be bitten by the same insects that bite IV addicts and sexually active individuals. In Belle Glade, the CDC said, AIDS was being spread mostly through contaminated needles or sexual activity, the same as elsewhere.

Inheritance
Given the fact that not everyone who has sex with an AIDS patient contracts the infection, that some individuals seem to be less susceptible to the disease, and that Africans seem to be more apt to get AIDS than American heterosexuals, it is not too farfetched to speculate that genetic factors may determine an individual's vulnerability. Scientists have known for some time that genes do play a part in how we react to certain infectious agents: hepatitis B, as mentioned, seems to be more infectious among Asians than among Westerners; and people without a certain blood factor are able to resist infection from one of the four types of malaria. There has been a long-standing suspicion that a similar genetic link would turn up in AIDS.

In June 1987, a team of British scientists turned up the first bit of evidence that genetic differences might influence individual susceptibility to the AIDS virus. Dr. Anthony A. Pinching and his colleagues at St. Mary's Hospital Medical School examined the blood of more than 200 individuals for a protein called group-specific component (Gc), which has three genetically determined variants. Those with one Gc type seemed to be protected against AIDS infection, while those with another type had a high incidence of the disease. Further testing is, of course, necessary before any strong conclusions can be drawn, and before the new data can lead — as some believe it will — to better treatment for AIDS.

11

Can AIDS Be Conquered?

Most men form an exaggerated estimate of the powers of medicine, founded on the common acceptance of the name, that medicine is the art of curing diseases. That this is a false definition is evident from the fact that many diseases are incurable, and that one such disease must at last happen to every living man. A far more just definition would be that medicine is the art of understanding diseases, and of curing and relieving them when possible.

— *Jacob Bigelow*

THE GAP IN TIME between identifying the cause of a disease like AIDS and finding a way to prevent, control, or eradicate it is often, unfortunately, a long one. It is true, of course, as Seneca once observed, that when a disease breaks forth from concealment and manifests its power, it is farther on the road to being cured. But the fact remains that virtually all of the infective agents that have plagued humankind down through the centuries have been as persistent in maintaining their grip on their hosts as the scientists have been in trying to loosen it.

The English country doctor Edward Jenner, for example, discovered in 1796 that inoculation with material from a cowpox lesion protected against the killer disease smallpox. He repeated the experiment two years later with identical results, published his findings, and predicted that vaccination (Jenner coined the term *vaccine* from the Latin for "cow," *vacca*) would eventually wipe out smallpox. But although vaccination soon after became compulsory in many European countries (some 100,000 persons, including Britain's royal family, were vaccinated worldwide by 1800), smallpox still continued to be a plague virtually everywhere, largely because global coordination and funds were lacking. As recently as 1967, an estimated 10 million to 15 million people contracted smallpox each year, and some 2 million perished. It was not until 1977, 181 years after Jenner's discovery, that the disease was at last exterminated.

Tuberculosis represents another case of lag between awareness of the disease and its control. The bacillus that causes TB, a disease that existed in Egypt as far back as 1000 B.C., was not positively identified until the German bacteriologist Robert Koch did so in 1882. It took two decades for prevailing medical opinion in the United States to accept his evidence that TB was not the result of an error in heredity, nor an exclusive affliction troubling only those of ethereal nature and languid pallor, but the result of an organism that could be passed from person to person. Not until 1944, with the discovery of streptomycin by Dr. Selman A. Waksman of Rutgers University, did researchers begin to feel they had taken a step toward effective chemotherapy for TB. Similarly, vaccination for polio, one of the most notable advances in preventive medicine, was used for the first time in the 1950s, some twenty years after researchers learned the disease was caused by a virus.

There is no reason to believe that the quest for an AIDS vaccine or an effective treatment will be any easier or take less time to realize. It is true that researchers today have access to knowledge and medical technology that an earlier generation of scientists could not even dream of. Jenner's vaccine was often sold on crude "vaccine points" — small quills with a coating of cowpox virus on the ends. And Koch did not even have access to a petri dish — the shallow, glass-covered culture dish in which bacteria are grown and that is among the most basic of today's laboratory equipment — until some five years after he discovered the TB bacillus.

But even with the current high state of the art of medical research, no one is predicting a quick solution to the AIDS outbreak. There is, at this writing, no treatment, and no vaccine. Nor will there soon be. (Considering that at least 115 viruses cause the common cold and, after years of trying, there is still no vaccine against any of them, that statement is not unfair.) In its most recent report, the Public Health Service said that no safe and effective treatment for AIDS can be expected "for the next several years," and no vaccine for widespread use to prevent infection can be expected "before the next decade."

What must be remembered is that AIDS is a viral infection, and while many infectious diseases caused by bacteria can be easily treated and controlled with antibiotics, those touched off by viruses are quite often another matter. Antibiotics are no good against any of them, and most treatments for viral diseases are limited to alleviating symptoms.

There are also some formidable obstacles to developing a vaccine to protect those not yet exposed to AIDS. The most difficult challenge seems to be overcoming virus variation, the ability of a virus to change its genetic structure, which, in turn, changes the very proteins in the envelope that would be targeted by a vaccine. Exactly why some viruses shift so drastically — and the AIDS virus seems to be able to change its colors as fast as the classic chameleon of the viral world, the flu virus — is unclear. It could be said that it evolves to protect itself, either by making itself invulnerable to different vaccines or by changing to a less dangerous form so it can hide, lying in wait for an opportune moment to strike. There is also the suspicion that just generating antibodies against the AIDS virus may not be enough to protect an individual (those who do make them appear to have extremely low levels).

And there is the matter of safety. Most antiviral vaccines, including those for polio, measles, and rubella, are made up of live viruses that have been attenuated, or weakened, enabling them to protect without causing the disease that bears their stamp. In the case of polio, two vaccines are in use: a live-virus vaccine that is administered orally, and an inactivated, or killed, virus vaccine that is injected. When these were first made available, they touched off considerable controversy over which was safer and more effective, and although some difference of opinion still exists, the oral vaccine is recommended by the World Health Organization's Expanded Program on Immunization and is more widely used. Given the lethality of the AIDS virus, however, some researchers are convinced that simply weakening it, as the polio virus is weakened when making the Sabin (oral) vaccine, is not an especially safe way to go since there is always the chance that it could regain its strength and start up the disease process. Even a "genetically killed" virus, one so altered that it theoretically cannot reproduce, could conceivably promote disease.

Nonetheless, researchers hunting for ways to treat or prevent AIDS, or both, are not deterred by the seemingly bleak outlook. For one thing, there are the proven vaccines against other, far-more-easily-transmitted viral diseases, like polio, flu, and measles; and two promising malaria vaccines are currently being tested. Even the chronic hepatitis B, caused by a virus that, as we have seen, is epidemiologically similar to the AIDS virus, may soon be weakening its hold. In July of 1986, the FDA gave its approval to a new hepatitis vaccine, the first genetically engineered one for human use; it can now be produced in great quantities, and is safer to use than the earlier vaccine, available since 1981, that is derived from the blood of patients infected with hepatitis.

Even the earlier vaccine seems to be effective in preventing uninfected people from getting hepatitis — and perhaps, ultimately, the liver cancer associated with the virus (even though relatively little is known about the relationship between hepatitis B and cancer). As Harvard's William Haseltine put it, "Even without a clue to the mechanism of how liver cancer arises in hepatitis-B carriers, we have the first effective cancer vaccine. If you eliminate the virus, you eliminate the disease. It's almost that simple." A handful of drugs that work against viral infections have also been developed and approved, among them acyclovir for general topical and oral use against herpesviruses; recent clinical studies have shown that a once-daily dose is even effective in preventing recurrent genital herpes.

Something else in the researchers' favor is the unprecedented wealth of information they have generated about AIDS, a feat that is nothing short of phenomenal, given the fact that the killer virus burst onto the scene relatively recently. The data have enabled scientists to grow the virus in the lab, disassemble its very genes, probe for its weak spots, identify precisely its mode of transmission and its potential victims, come up with a highly accurate test to detect exposure to the virus and block its spread through the supply of blood and blood products, and improve the treatments aimed at the specific diseases that AIDS patients get.

And so an air of "cautious optimism," that overworked term used by scientists, prevails in the laboratories. Currently, researchers are concentrating their efforts in three areas in the fight against AIDS: (1) finding ways to restore or augment the disarmed immune systems of victims; (2) finding drugs that will halt the growth of the virus (thus stopping it from spreading cell to cell) and that can be used to treat the opportunistic disorders and various symptoms that accompany AIDS-virus infection; and (3) finding a vaccine. Here is a rundown of the research work aimed in those directions.

IMMUNOMODULATION

It seems logical, given the AIDS virus's penchant for attacking and overwhelming the very cells the body marshals to defend itself against foreign substances, that by strengthening the immune system — by rearming and retraining it, as it were, and goading it into facing up to the deadly virus — the disease might well be controlled.

In early 1987, there was, in fact, some encouraging evidence that this might be possible. Jay Levy and his team at the University of California at San Francisco reported that suppressor T-cells appear to be able to control the AIDS virus in cell culture and, evidently, in some patients, leading to the conclusion that a patient's own immune system can fight the virus without the use of antiviral drugs. Levy began by studying a specific subset of individuals infected with the AIDS virus who had no signs of the disease, nor any trace of the virus in their blood. Half of all healthy but antibody-positive people, according to Levy, fall into this group, and some of those he has followed for a year have shown improvements in their immune systems.

To try to find out why the immune systems in these people are apparently able to control the virus and prevent it from reproducing, Levy and his colleagues took blood samples from three healthy homosexual men — men who had antibodies to the virus but no detectable virus in their blood — and removed the suppressor T-cells. The results were dramatic: the virus began to grow in the samples that had been stripped of their suppressor cells, indicating that the cells had been blocking reproduction of the virus; when the cells were put back into the blood samples, replication of the AIDS virus was once again suppressed.

"This is the first indication," said Levy, "that individuals have in themselves a means of controlling the virus. This discovery could be the first step toward an effective therapy for AIDS, using a person's own immune cells rather than drugs that are toxic to the body."[1] Added Christopher Walker, a principal investigator in the study: "It shows that if you are infected with the virus, you don't necessarily have to get the disease — your immune system can fight it off." The findings also support the theory proposed earlier by Levy that AIDS is an opportunistic infection itself, one that will cause disease only in someone whose immune system has been severely weakened in some way, as by a chronic infection.

The findings are, of course, heartening. But other researchers urged caution in jumping from the test tube to the living patient. So far, the approaches that seem to work best are those that combine immunologic reconstitution with antiviral therapy.

Bone Marrow Transplants
This surgical procedure, actually a transfusion, was developed as an adjunct to chemotherapy and radiation for leukemia, a malignant disease in which the patient's bone marrow churns out huge quantities of abnormal white blood cells and platelets, causing anemia, bleeding disorders, and, as in AIDS, a lowering of the body's natural defenses against infection. (The analogy between AIDS and leukemia cannot, however, be carried far.

In the case of the blood malignancy, the leukemia virus HTLV-I causes helper T-cells to proliferate wildly. The related AIDS virus has the opposite effect: it destroys the T-cells.)

Some 800 marrow grafts are performed each year in the United States, approximately 3,000 worldwide. In 1986, the most desperately ill victims of the Chernobyl nuclear accident in the Soviet Union received either bone marrow or marrow substitute extracted from the livers of aborted fetuses (embryonic liver is the major site for the production of blood cells) in an effort to restore immune systems devastated by exposure to high doses of radiation.

The procedure is relatively simple. With a special syringe and needle, and while the donor is under general anesthesia, about two pints of marrow, in clear liquid form and containing a billion cells, are drawn from the donor's pelvic bone, purified, and introduced into the recipient's bloodstream through an intravenous line. (Marrow cells replenish themselves quickly, and the amount removed is generally replaced in two to three weeks.) Once in the bloodstream of the recipient, the marrow migrates to the interior of the major bones, and soon produces healthy, new blood cells.

The success of the procedure depends on the genetic closeness of donor and recipient, with identical twins or siblings considered the best donors. Even subtle differences in genetic matching can put the immune system's surveillance mechanism on alert, resulting in an attack being mounted against the transplanted marrow tissue. Still, some 50 percent to 60 percent of recipients survive for at least a year, and marrow grafting has taken its place as an important, though still developing, means of treating at least fifteen diseases other than leukemia. Among them are lymphomas, multiple myeloma, a number of solid tumors, and several genetic and immune-system disorders such as SCID (for "severe combined immunodeficiency"), which, like AIDS, severely impairs its victims' defenses.

The most celebrated use of a marrow transplant to treat SCID involved the case of David, the so-called Bubble-Boy, who because of his immune deficiency, spent all but a few days of his twelve years of life in a plastic, germ-free "bubble." His doctors, in a desperate attempt to bolster his defenses enough to enable him to leave his protective chamber, decided on a marrow graft from David's sister. It was unsuccessful. David died in a Houston hospital in February 1984, of a lymphatic cancer believed to have been caused by an Epstein-Barr virus transported into his body in the donor marrow.

Like SCID, AIDS, because of its devastating effect on the immune system, would seem to be a prime candidate for treatment by bone marrow transplantation, which provides the body with an instant source of immune cells. But although in theory the procedure is attractive, and technically a fairly simple one, its application to AIDS patients has not generally met with success. It was tried, in fact, before the AIDS virus was even identified, in an infected homosexual male who received healthy marrow taken from his identical, heterosexual, twin brother. In that case, reported by Dr. Anthony Fauci, head of the National Institute of Allergy and Infectious Diseases, there was a temporary, minor improvement in immunologic function in the form of a delayed-type hypersensitivity skin reaction, and an increase in the number of T-4 lymphocytes. The patient eventually died of a number of opportunistic infections and fast-moving Kaposi's sarcoma. Because the trial came before the virus had been identified, no antiviral treatment was possible.

To date, there has been one notable AIDS success with bone marrow transplantation: an AIDS patient in his early thirties who received a novel combination of bone marrow transplant from his identical twin brother, treatment with the antiviral drug suramin (a long-popular drug used to treat parasitic diseases such as African sleeping sickness), and transfusions of lymphocyte blood cells. At this writing, the patient was in apparently good health a year after treatment, recovered enough to return to full-time work. Posttreatment examination has revealed dramatic increases in his T-4 cells, a shrinking to normal of swollen lymph nodes (in which Kaposi's sarcoma had been detected earlier), and no evidence of the AIDS virus in his blood. Commenting on the case, Fauci cautioned that while it clearly established the feasibility of the technique in reconstituting an AIDS-depleted immune system, "long-term follow-up would be required to determine whether the patient's immune function will be maintained and/or continue to improve and whether the retrovirus will be contained."[2]

Thus far, only a few other patients have received marrow transfers — all from their identical twin brothers — and though there was some improvement in immune function, the course of the disease was not affected, probably because the virus was still in the body. In the one successful transplant case just described, Fauci has pointed out, the likelihood exists that the patient is still actively infected with the virus since it is clear that the drug, suramin, has not been effective in suppressing the AIDS virus in a living organism. (Two other patients were given the combination treatment, but it failed in both instances.)

Also, while transplanted marrow begins to repopulate the patient's immune system with healthy cells about two weeks after the procedure, for three to four weeks there simply are not enough mature cells to ward off all kinds of previously inactive disease organisms, let alone something so relentless and stealthy as the AIDS virus. In fact, marrow transplant patients are generally advised not to return to work or school for six to nine months after the procedure, even though blood tests appear to be normal, because the immune system needs time to recover. And again, so long as the AIDS virus remains in a patient's body, he is in jeopardy, especially during recuperation from a marrow transplant, when close to a year of convalescence, physically and emotionally, is required because the immune system is in such a weakened state.

The bottom line of all of this is that while there has been an apparent, significant beneficial effect on the immune system and suppression of the virus in one of three patients who received a combination of bone marrow transplant and other modalities, this form of treatment for AIDS is still in its infancy. Even if bone marrow taken from matched relatives other than identical twins is tried in patients with the disease, it will, unfortunately, be a long time before the treatment becomes routine.

Biological-Response Modifiers
Much touted lately as potential anticancer agents, these types of protein substances, known scientifically as lymphokines (from

lymphocyte and the Greek *kinen,* for "to move"), help carry out many of the functions of the T-4 lymphocytes. Produced in small amounts when white cells are challenged by foreign substances, such as cancer cells and viruses, the lymphokines travel from cell to cell, carrying a message through the immune system telling it how to deal with the threat. They can now be produced in large quantities through genetic engineering. Several show early promise against AIDS and, according to scientists like Fauci, deserve further investigation.

Perhaps the best known is interferon, now approved for commercial use as a cancer drug. Drawing its name from its ability to interfere with the reproduction of viruses, it was discovered in 1957 by Alick Isaacs and Jean Lindemann, of the National Institute of Medical Research in London, who noticed that the cells of chick embryos infected with influenza released a mysterious substance. When they added it to other cells, the cells became resistant to the flu virus.

Researchers later found that this interferon had antitumor properties as well as antiviral ones. When interferon is injected into the body, it can attack cancers and interfere with their metabolism, or it encourages T- and B-cells and macrophages to destroy them.

Interferons come in three major forms: alpha, beta, and gamma. Humans carry at least twelve genes that make alpha-interferon, a form produced by B-lymphocytes, and because the genes have different nucleic-acid sequences, each product they produce is unique. By contrast, there is one human beta-interferon gene, and one gamma-interferon gene.

Gamma-interferon, which was tried on AIDS patients at the NIH from February 1983 to September 1984, has come out the loser. In one study, when it was injected into patients in a wide range of doses, there were no clinical benefits even at the highest dose range. Side effects at the higher doses (hepatitis, fever, and nausea) were also so pronounced that the trial at those levels had to be halted.

Alpha-interferon may be another story. In June of 1986, it won FDA approval as the first commercial cancer treatment developed by the genetic-engineering industry. Although the drug is approved only for treatment of hairy-cell leukemia (the rare disease that must usually be treated by removing the spleen), against which it has induced complete or partial remissions in up to 90 percent of the patients treated, there are indications it is also effective against genital warts, hepatitis B, the common cold, and — of special interest to AIDS researchers — Kaposi's sarcoma.

Studies have shown, in fact, that alpha-interferon induced either partial or complete regression of Kaposi's lesions in some AIDS patients, especially when the lesions were not extensive and where immune functions were not severely suppressed. In one trial at Memorial Sloan-Kettering Cancer Center in New York City, alpha-interferon induced long-lasting regressions of Kaposi's sarcoma, along with a degree of preservation of immune function, in one-fourth of 91 patients; the median duration for complete responders was 24 months, and for partial responders, 11.5 months. Five of the complete responders were free of the disease 31 to 44 months after treatment was stopped. Moreover, according to Dr. Susan E. Krown, an associate attending physician at the center, there were indications that interferon may also have prevented the virus from causing infection in the bloodstream — the first clinical evidence that the drug may inhibit the AIDS virus.[3]

Despite the relatively positive results, the researchers emphasized that their data were still preliminary. "The numbers are very small," said Dr. Loretta Itri, director of clinical oncology at Hoffmann–La Roche, makers of the interferon. "We don't have a historical group of patients to compare the trial group with, and we can't even say with certainty at this point whether these patients represent a subset that was inadvertently selected, or whether in fact we are witnessing a true, interferon-related phenomenon."[4] Krown added that many Kaposi's patients do well on conventional chemotherapy without serious side effects, but pointed out a difference: with conventional treatment, there is little reason to believe that chemotherapy has any effect on anything but the tumor; but with interferon, there is at least the hope that when patients respond there may be beneficial effects on the underlying disease.[5]

Another of the biological-response modifiers that show some

promise against AIDS is interleukin-2 (IL-2), an immune-system activator that, when synthesized and mixed with lymphocytes in the lab, then experimentally injected into a cancer patient along with more interleukin, can transform the lymphocytes into cancer killers that attack the malignancy but spare most normal tissue. Recently, the treatment was used to shrink tumors by about 50 percent in 11 of 25 severely ill patients with lung, kidney, colon, and skin cancer; in 1, the tumor regressed completely. (Subsequent tests with the drug did not, however, produce the same heartening results, and in one recent study, the success rates ranged between 10 percent and 30 percent.)

Based on interleukin's potential, scientists began testing it in AIDS patients with Kaposi's sarcoma. Preliminary results indicated that the drug does enhance the lymphocyte count and causes a reduction, albeit a fairly minor one, in the size of Kaposi's tumors in some patients. Neither of the effects, however, brought about any significant clinical improvement in the patients. Nonetheless, Fauci's group has continued to use interleukin-2 in over 50 patients. "The results are promising," he has reported, "and as with alpha-interferon, serious consideration will be given to using IL-2 in combination with an anti-retroviral agent and/or another immunomodulator."[6]

An interesting, little-known sidelight to the interleukin story, and one that may have some clinical value in preventing the insidious progression from infection to AIDS, recently emerged from research at the George Washington University Medical Center. There, biochemist Allan Goldstein — codiscoverer of the thymosins, hormones produced by the thymus that play a role in controlling immunity — has found that low-dose aspirin can increase the production of interleukin-2 and that this new immune-modulating role for the popular analgesic may increase the effectiveness of biological-response modifiers, such as thymosin, in treating a wide range of diseases linked to a malfunctioning, thymus-dependent immune system, among them AIDS, rheumatoid arthritis, and lung cancer.

Goldstein's first clinical trials began with thymosin injections in individuals in early stages of AIDS. Although there were some encouraging results both in immune function and in sustaining the health of the patients, there was no significant improvement on a cellular level — until Goldstein added aspirin and tried the mixture out on normal volunteers and in the test tube. When he combined aspirin with thymosin, he found a significant increase in interleukin-2 over that seen with thymosin alone. "Aspirin alone," says Goldstein,

> shows a distinct ability to markedly increase the output of interleukin-2 and may also affect other growth factors produced by the immune system necessary for developing resistance to viruses and cancer. Stimulating the immune system with a combination of thymosins and aspirin may make a significant difference in preventing progression to AIDS and improve both survival and quality of life for individuals at risk for AIDS. We know a great deal about the actions of both thymosins and aspirin when given separately, and now we have a strong rationale to study their effectiveness in combination for patients at risk for AIDS.[7]

Clinical trials to further test Goldstein's theory are currently under way among at-risk patients. By measuring improvements in immune function — enhanced production of the body's antiviral agents, and the capacity of patients to prevent subsequent infection — researchers should be able to learn if the new approach has any merit.

Even if interleukin does not pan out as an AIDS therapy per se, its very presence in the body of a patient may signal which patients can be treated with it. Dr. Charles Kirkpatrick of the National Jewish Hospital and Research Center in Denver has found, for example, that AIDS patients with opportunistic infections, and those with Kaposi's sarcoma along with such infections, fail to produce interleukin-2. But AIDS patients who have only Kaposi's do. The finding is significant because interleukin-2 mediates interferon production, and failure to produce interleukin may well be an additional abnormality that predisposes AIDS patients to opportunistic infections.

Several other possible ways to shore up failed immune systems are also being explored, among them:

• IMREG-I. Manufactured by Imreg, Inc., of New Orleans, this immune modulator derived from white blood cells appears to enhance the production of other biological-response modifiers, such as interleukin-2 and gamma-interferon. Preliminary tests in patients with mild forms of AIDS, and ARC, showed some improvement, and the drug was being tested at this writing in 150 patients at a number of medical centers.

• GM-CSF. This new biological-response modifier is a genetically engineered human-growth hormone. In preliminary trials during the past year, researchers were able to increase production of some white blood cells by manipulating the dosage of the hormone. The hormone, which does not stimulate T-4 cells, has been tried on 16 AIDS patients. It forced their other white-cell counts way up, providing a few patients who had had no immune responses with fairly strong ones. Researchers hope the therapy will be useful against the opportunistic infections that accompany AIDS.

• Gamma globulin. Made naturally in the body and containing antibodies to infections, this substance gives temporary, or passive, immunity when injected into someone who has been exposed to an infection under some circumstances, such as might occur in a local epidemic of measles. The antibodies, however, are depleted fairly quickly, and immunity lasts only as long as they are present in the blood, usually a few weeks. In general, this form of immunization is helpful if administered before symptoms appear.

Immunoglobulin therapy is currently under investigation in the treatment of infants with AIDS, a group whose plight is magnified by the fact that their immune systems are destroyed before they have been able to fully develop. Such children are prey to all manner of opportunistic infections, many of them fatal. Not long ago, scientists at Albert Einstein College of Medicine in New York City reported they had treated 14 AIDS infants with intravenous injections of gamma globulin over a three-year period. Although the treatment had no effect on the AIDS itself, the results were heartening: only 3 cases of fever lasting more than a week, and 1 episode of circulatory-system infection, all the result of bacterial infections and common among children with AIDS.

By contrast, all but 1 of 27 AIDS children who did not receive gamma globulin contracted fevers that lasted more than a week, and most of them worsened or died. (None of the treated children died during the study period, but at this writing, 8 had.) While pointing out that gamma globulin treatment only temporarily shored up the children's defenses, the doctors, nonetheless, felt that it seemed to enhance the quality of the children's lives by staving off the added misery of additional infections.

• Cyclosporine. Credited with dramatically improving the survival rate of transplant patients by preventing the rejection of organ grafts, this drug seems a paradoxical way to treat AIDS. It is an immunosuppressor, an agent that depresses the immune system so that it does not recognize the transplanted organ as foreign. Most of the other approaches, as we have seen, try to restore and boost immune function, not relegate the immune system to the category of an undesirable side effect. They are, of course, based on the widely held belief that the AIDS virus directly attacks the cells of the immune system (among others); thus, anything that might aid and abet that attack — drugs like cyclosporine, for instance — would place the patient further in jeopardy by opening the way for more infections.

But there is another theory, a controversial one held by several researchers, among them scientists at the Laennec Hospital in Paris, where cyclosporine has been tested, thus far, on 23 AIDS patients. It suggests that somehow the AIDS virus tricks the immune system into attacking and destroying itself — the phenomenon known as autoimmunity.

The French are not alone in holding on to the autoimmunity theory. In a recent paper in the journal *Clinical Immunology and Immunopathology,* Dr. John Ziegler and Dr. Daniel Stites of the University of California at San Francisco (UCSF) questioned the premise that AIDS develops because the virus invades and kills white blood cells that normally marshal the body's immune defenses. "We are," said Ziegler, "among a small but growing group of skeptics who think it's not that simple, because what you see in the early stages of AIDS isn't an immune deficiency but an immune system in overdrive."[8]

Even when the disease was recognized in 1981, he pointed out, doctors found that patients at first displayed swollen lymph nodes, high levels of antibodies — including some against normal tissue such as blood platelets — and other signs of a distracted defense system. Damage to skin, the central nervous system, joints, kidneys, and other organs often mimicked that seen in some of the autoimmune diseases or graft-versus-host reactions in organ transplant patients. Then, numbers of T-helper cells and certain other cells gradually dropped, and the rare cancers or infections occurred. Such phenomena could not be explained by viral multiplication alone, Ziegler maintained, noting that even in later stages of the disease, the virus can be found in only about 1 of 10,000 helper lymphocytes.

The UCSF team believes, instead, that the virus triggers AIDS by mimicking certain kinds of "self" markers found on many cells of the immune system — markers that help identify the cells as a legitimate part of that person. As the body mounts an attack against the virus, the antibodies and attacking cells might confuse the virus with the self-markers. "So by mistake, the immune system would be waging war against its own soldiers," says Ziegler. "This mutinous situation would result in a progressive drop in innocent bystander cells with these particular self markers — including T-cells, B-cells and macrophages — until the whole system burned out. And as AIDS progresses, that's exactly what we see."[9]

There are several bona fide examples of autoimmune disease. In rheumatoid arthritis, the immune system attacks and destroys linings around the joints, viewing the target as "nonself." In systemic lupus erythematosus (SLE, or lupus), the immune system turns against the body's connective tissues and kidneys with a variety of autoantibodies (abnormal antibodies against the body's own tissues). Type I diabetes is believed to result when the insulin-producing islet cells in the pancreas are destroyed by an immune response.

If AIDS falls into this category of diseases (and so far the burden of proof appears to be on those who suggest that it does), then the use of cyclosporine is logical. Because it works by holding off the immune system's efforts to wipe out a foreign substance, as it does when it is used to restrain the system from rejecting a transplanted organ, it could — if, indeed, AIDS is an autoimmune disorder in which the virus forces the victim's defenses to turn inward — block that bizarre process. It would do this, the theory goes, by blocking stimulation and duplication of T-cells already infected with the AIDS virus. The uninfected cells would, thus, continue to replicate, and the immune system would rebuild itself. Since even increases in other immune cells might offer some protection against the fatal opportunistic infections that accompany AIDS, patients would benefit. "If autoimmunity plays a major role," says Ziegler, "it makes sense that at an early stage in AIDS, the self-destruction could be brought in check."[10]

When French doctors first announced, at a hastily called news conference in October of 1985, that they had produced "dramatic" improvement in two AIDS patients after only a week of treatment with cyclosporine, they were roundly criticized for their premature judgment. (Another patient in the end stages of AIDS had also been treated with cyclosporine, for two days, and had died before the news conference.) The French have opted to continue their research with cyclosporine, arguing now that while it clearly does not work in those already diagnosed with AIDS, it may block the disease in those who have pre-AIDS — that is, those individuals who do not have symptoms, but who have antibodies to the virus.

The use of cyclosporine, thus, seems to have some merit, especially when one considers that substances like interleukin-2 may merely create a larger pool of virus-replicating T-cells. But cyclosporine is not without its drawbacks. One is, of course, that it might help an otherwise healthy individual contract some serious ailments (again, infection with the AIDS virus does not necessarily mean the person will get AIDS). Immunosuppressive drugs can also have severe side effects and be difficult to control. In fact, transplant patients who have been given cyclosporine and later contracted AIDS through a contaminated blood transfusion have not done well. The best treatments, says Ziegler, would selectively suppress the attacking cells, while allowing more protective responses to remain intact.

• Isoprinosine. A chemically synthesized immune-system modulator, this drug was originally developed in the 1970s to enhance memory in the elderly. In one study conducted at St. Luke's–Roosevelt Hospital in New York City with a small number of patients with AIDS and related illnesses, the drug failed to demonstrate any clinical benefit. In another test of 157 ARC patients, the drug was said to have improved immune function in 110. But, according to the FDA, claims made by the manufacturer, Newport Pharmaceuticals International, Inc., were unfounded. The FDA has said that the firm's data showed only a small effect on one of the many types of immunoactive cells, and no consistent effect on any other element of the immune system. Furthermore, according to the FDA, studies the company said showed a 50-percent reduction in the progression rate of ARC to full-scale AIDS were too small to produce meaningful conclusions. The agency also notified the firm that its promotion of therapeutic claims for isoprinosine might constitute promotion of an unapproved drug and thus would violate the Food, Drug and Cosmetic Act.

• Lymphotoxin. Not something that one administers to a patient, this is a natural protein substance that researchers are, instead, trying to remove from the immune system in the hope that doing so will halt the progression of AIDS. Lymphotoxins are normally produced by white blood cells to fight tumor cells, viruses, and germs, but when they are produced in very high quantities, as they might be in AIDS, they may cause a cell to self-destruct. Interfering with a virus-infected cell's production of the protein, thus, might be a way to treat AIDS, because instead of trying to restore T-cells after they are killed, the focus would be on the mechanism that destroys the cells in the first place.

Such therapy is still hypothesis, and was only recently suggested by Yale microbiologist Nancy Ruddle, who has admitted her evidence is "midway between suggestive and sure."[11] Although the mechanism by which the AIDS virus induces lymphotoxin is not known, it is suggested that the virus could stimulate it directly, or that it might trigger high levels of interleukin-2, which then activates production. Also unclear is whether lymphotoxin turns against the very cells that produced it, or against other nearby T- cells. It may well be, as Ruddle observes, that "too much lymphotoxin is made and the body doesn't need it. Because no target exists to absorb it, it feeds back on the cells and kills them off."[12]

Ruddle believes that lymphotoxins — which inhibit an enzyme essential to lipid metabolism, and thus disturb the digestion of certain foods, notably fats — may cause several characteristics of AIDS, such as reduced body weight and a smaller number of circulating T-cells. Thus far, she has tested the serum of 12 AIDS patients for lymphotoxin content, turning up the destructive protein in 8 of them. Moreover, in laboratory cultures, she found that uninfected T-cells from non-AIDS patients contained very little lymphotoxin, but that when cells were infected with the AIDS virus, production of the protein was dramatically increased, with the peak output coming before the cells died.

If her hypothesis proves correct, Ruddle sees two ways of perhaps reversing the deadly course of AIDS. One would be to inhibit lymphotoxin production, either by using a specially tailored antibody, or perhaps cyclosporine, or by chemically binding the lymphotoxin so it does not feed back on the T- cells and kill them. Another useful method might be to block the receptor, the site of attachment, for lymphotoxin in the T-cell. "If you understand what components make up the receptor," Ruddle explains, "then you can actually present the patient with those components in a high enough quantity to compete with the receptor for lymphotoxin."[13] The receptors have already been shown to contain certain sugars to which lymphotoxins will bind, so with an understanding of the protein structure of the receptor, agents could be introduced to stop the lymphotoxin from binding to the receptor and killing the cell.

• Psychoneuroimmunology and vitamins. No discussion of manipulating the body's natural defenses is complete without at least mention of the link between the immune and the nervous systems, and the effects of fitness, diet, and stress on our immune responses. For years, scientists have known that the vital immunological organs and tissues — the thymus, bone marrow, and lymph nodes — are joined with nerve fibers that originate in the brain, and that if they destroyed or stimulated portions of an experimental animal's brain, they could boost its ability to fight infection, or suppress it. They also know that various brain chemicals can force immune cells to multiply, and that brain-secreted hormones can also affect the way the body fights disease.

All of this is evidence, for many researchers who pursue the new science of psychoneuroimmunology, that the mind, indeed, is involved in manipulating our immunological defense system, and that the immune system can be turned on and off, in a sense, at will, or unwittingly. And so, many researchers say they have come up with evidence to prove that positive thinking, a healthy attitude, and mental imagery that focuses on actually battling a disease like, say, cancer can be used successfully to fight off the disease and improve survival. They know, also, that grief can temporarily injure immune function, and there is mounting evidence that daily, garden-variety stresses, as well as heavier pressures, can alter the level of T-cells just enough to set off a wide range of disorders from allergies to genital herpes.

Insofar as AIDS is concerned, some specialists have suggested that it could have a connection to psychoneuroimmunology. Its victims often develop severe depression, which, in turn, may endanger the immune system and thereby further suppress it. The emotional stress may also worsen AIDS-related dementia. Because of such associations, the National Institute of Mental Health has already committed several million dollars to study the behavioral aspects of AIDS.

It should be obvious, too, given the vital connection between what we eat and our health, that poor diet certainly does not nourish the cells that shore up our natural defenses against disease. Neither does lack of exercise, for physical exertion stimulates the production and increases the efficiency of immune cells. Factors other than viruses, then, can and do create a malfunctioning or deficient immune system.

Certainly, because so little is known about the connection between mind, disease, and immunological changes, no AIDS treatment program can rely solely on behavior modification or a change in diet as an effective way to prod the immune system into dealing with the disease. But, as was pointed out earlier in this book, various cofactors, among them poor hygiene and malnutrition, may very well play a role in whether and how AIDS gains a foothold. Correcting some of these problems, therefore, might help prevent or even treat an infection with the AIDS virus.

In light of how very little can actually be done for an AIDS patient, and because no immunorestorative agent has yet been discovered that completely corrects the underlying defect that makes AIDS what it is, nonmedical means cannot and should not be discounted or discouraged, for they may well help. They will do no harm so long as they are not expensive therapy scams — and many vulnerable AIDS patients are, indeed, being ripped off by scams that deny the virus-caused nature of the disease and blame it, as some pseudopractitioners have, on imbalances between yin and yang, or on guilt, anxiety, sweets, and fatty foods. Overreliance on such specious supports can cause an AIDS patient to delay conventional therapy that may help treat some of the illnesses that often accompany an AIDS infection.

But AIDS patients, those with the disease itself and with related conditions, might test the effects of a macrobiotic diet, and perhaps vitamin and mineral supplements, to see if these measures do help them feel better and maybe even repair some of the damage already done. A report not long ago in *Medical World News* noted that a year after converting to a macrobiotic diet, 24 Kaposi's patients in one study "showed stabilized percentages of T-4 helper cells and had total lymphocyte counts within normal ranges." Although 6 of the 24 died, the average survival has been more than two years — comparable to any other AIDS treatment. "What's exciting," the report quoted biochemist John Beldekas of Boston University as saying, "is that a conservative treatment seems to stabilize immune function, as opposed to drug treatments that often knock out immune function."[14]

Vitamin C, too, may have a place. Long touted by scientists like Linus Pauling, who downs 10,000 milligrams of it a day (the official recommended daily allowance ranges from 35 to 75 milligrams), ascorbic acid allegedly helps fight off the common cold and, according to one study with advanced cancer patients, conducted by Pauling, led to a fourfold increase in their life expectancy. That vitamim C has a role to play in many biological processes, including a central one in the proper functioning of both the nervous and endocrine systems, is fairly well established.

The aforementioned issue of *Medical World News* also carried a report on the work of a California orthopedic surgeon, Robert F. Cathcart III, who strongly believes that a take-charge attitude, combined with heavy doses of vitamin C and regular exercise, can protect and boost an AIDS patient's immune system. At the time of the report, Cathcart had treated more than 100 Kaposi's patients with up to 200 grams a day of vitamin C (the toxicity of AIDS, he says, brings about an acute form of scurvy that requires that the vitamin be forced into tissues), along with high doses of zinc, selenium, manganese, and vitamins A and E; 20 of the patients were in remission, and 80 had survived an average of three years. Also, 20 pneumocystosis patients treated with vitamin C plus sulfa were in remission, and a few patients with ARC had a doubling of their T-cells.

Unconventional therapies do have their place in AIDS treatment, even though relatively little is known about them. The intricate chemical-communication system that is strung between substances produced by the disease-fighting white blood cells and those produced by nerve cells in the brain may well mean that the brain is, in a sense, talking to the immune system. If that chemical conversation includes a message from the brain to the effect that, "Listen, this brain is thinking positive, so marshal your defenses and maybe you'll beat this thing, or at least feel better," then for the AIDS or the ARC patient, it is worth a try.

DRUGS

Hope, it is true, is about all an AIDS patient has to hold on to. Sometimes, it is the hope that the terrible disease will miraculously disappear through some holistic alternative to medicines — a hope, unfortunately, that rarely if ever is realized, since miracles, like lottery hits, work on long odds.

Many patients, however, are counting on some new drug, or an old one tailored to new purpose, in hopes that it will rid their bodies of the ravaging virus. That expectation, edged with urgency, is shared by a legion of researchers here and abroad. Recently, this appeal appeared in an advertisement in the journal *Science:*

> The National Cancer Institute and the National Institute of Allergy and Infectious Diseases of the NIH have jointly organized an AIDS Drug Selection Committee to review and facilitate the development [testing] of possible treatments for AIDS. This committee is constituted to review suggestions submitted for treatment of AIDS patients and, in certain cases, to recommend appropriate pre-clinical and clinical research or further development. Interested parties who have synthetic or natural substances known to inhibit the growth of the retrovirus known to cause AIDS, or which may preserve or augment the immune status of infected persons, are encouraged to share that information.

In June 1986, NIH widened its search for a drug to treat AIDS by funding controlled studies of promising drugs; five-year contracts totaling $100 million went to fourteen medical centers throughout the United States. The drugs likely to be used first included the immunity-enhancer alpha-interferon and several antivirals, among them azidothymidine (AZT), Foscarnet, HPA-23, ribavirin, and dideoxycytidine (DDC). At this writing, trials were under way, and if one or more of the drugs seems to show more promise, the trials will be expanded.

But developing and testing promising drugs against AIDS does not, of course, guarantee success. The history of medicine is replete with tales of potentially useful treatments that turned out to be either useless or harmful. Thalidomide, a supposedly harmless sleeping pill widely used in West Germany some years ago, comes immediately to mind. The drug was eventually withdrawn from the market after doctors began reporting cases of grotesquely malformed babies born to mothers who had taken it during early pregnancy. Cancer drugs are another example. Every year between 1955 and 1975, thousands of agents potentially useful against cancer cells were tested; but of the thirty or so drugs currently available, most came out of the laboratories between 1940 and 1965, and of those thirty or so, only a handful are considered mainstays in fighting cancer. They are also hardly an unmitigated blessing: when they work, they bring about dramatic results; when they are bad, as they so frequently are, their side effects are devastating as they shoot through the body in scattergun fashion, killing healthy cells as well as cancerous ones.

Chemotherapy has worked well against acute lymphocytic leukemia, markedly increasing the cure rate among children, and it has had a few successes in some tumors that are hard to treat, like lung and (when combined with radiotherapy) pancreatic cancer; reviews of breast cancer studies also show that chemotherapy and hormonal therapy can be effective in reducing the number of deaths from that disease; and early drug treatment has had some effect on rectal, head, and neck cancers. But the drugs are still inefficient in treating carcinomas, the tumors that constitute 80 percent to 90 percent of all malignancies and that originate in the epithelial tissue, which makes up the skin and lines all hollow organs of the respiratory, digestive, and urinary systems.

If drug inefficiency seems to come with the territory with such a long-known and widespread disease as cancer, it is highly unlikely that any immediate cures for AIDS, about which there is still much to learn, will emerge soon from the laboratory. That statement is admittedly a pessimistic one, and a difficult one for a science writer, who generally tries to find hope in any medical story, to make. But it should not be taken to mean that researchers must stop trying to find a drug treatment; drugs, after all, do work, and wonderfully so, and they have been responsible for saving countless millions from death and disability.

But AIDS, once again, is a peculiar disease, and finding an effective drug to wipe it out is no easy job for many reasons, some of which were noted earlier. One is, of course, the virus's ability to commandeer the synthesizing, inner machinery of the cell it has invaded, becoming such an intimate part of the now-captive cell that any drugs aimed at the virus stand a good chance of knocking out the cell as well. An attempt to get at the AIDS virus, barricaded as it were by the plasma membrane of the cell, is thus somewhat akin to trying to kill a hostage-taker in a fortified building without killing or injuring the hostages.

There are other stumbling blocks. One was thrown in the way by the discovery that the AIDS virus can also take cellular hostages in the brain. An anti-AIDS drug would have to cross the blood-brain barrier, the formidable wall of tightly packed cells lining the capillaries of the central nervous system that quite effectively insulates the brain from bacteria and other potentially dangerous agents traveling through the bloodstream. But the barrier can be too efficient. Some drugs cannot get through the tiny spaces between the cells, while others are only able to trickle through. Because of this hindrance, drugs must often be given in frequent, extremely high doses in order to achieve even the minimum concentration effective in the brain. But such heavy blood levels of these limited-access drugs can damage other organs, especially the liver and kidneys, and a number of conditions simply cannot be treated easily. Among these are brain tumors, bacterial or viral infections such as meningitis, and infection of the central nervous system by the AIDS virus.

Several approaches to breaching the barrier are, however, being tested. One novel method that may have some eventual application to AIDS has been developed by Dr. Nicholas Bodor, a medicinal chemist at the University of Florida. His system utilizes a "carrier" molecule that is capable of assuming both fat and water-soluble forms. When a drug is chemically linked to the carrier, the drug becomes much more soluble than in its original form and is able to slip much more easily through the blood-brain barrier; inside the brain, naturally occurring enzymes reconvert the drug-loaded molecule to a water-soluble state and its exit is thus blocked by the barrier. With the drug complex trapped in brain tissue, another enzyme gradually releases the drug, giving it time to exert its therapeutic effect.

Another hindrance to developing an AIDS drug or a vaccine is the battleground on which the virus has chosen to make its stand. No other infectious disease in history, not even the plague or polio, specifically targets the body's immune system as its victim. For that reason alone, AIDS researchers lack a precedent for devising a drug that not only kills the virus and preserves cellular integrity but also restores the ravaged immune system. Any effort to accomplish such an enormous feat would, in light of current knowledge, have to be put on a back burner while researchers concentrate on finding the right combination of antiviral agent and immune booster, just as they have had to come up with the most effective combinations of anticancer drugs.

Roland K. Robins, director of molecular research at Nucleic Acid Research Institute of Costa Mesa, California, lists several criteria that antiviral drugs should meet if they are to be effective.[15] They are indeed demanding (even more so when applied to a newer disease like AIDS):

- The drug should exert broad-spectrum activity, since in many cases it still is not easy to identify specific viruses from clinical specimens.
- The drug should have sufficient potency for complete inhibition of viral replication. Incomplete inhibition may only prolong the disease.
- The drug should not suppress normal processes that develop active immunity in the patient. In the ideal case, the antiviral agent may hold the virus in check while the immune system gears up to finish the job of eliminating the last virus.
- The drug should not be susceptible to the emergence of resistant viral variants. Such resistance is still a problem when treating bacterial infections with antibiotics.
- Finally, as mentioned earlier, the drug should have a minimum toxicity for the host cell.

Investigators testing nearly a core of anti-AIDS drugs add that the ideal one would also be orally administered, would cross the blood-brain barrier, would be nontoxic, and would produce its effect with a limited course of therapy. Criteria are, however, one thing, and meeting them quite another. It is no laboratory piece of cake to come up with a potent yet safe drug that must inhibit reverse transcriptase, the specific enzyme that the virus uses to reproduce itself, so as to interfere in the replication process (the presumed goal of most antiviral agents investigated to date); or perhaps that must change the membrane of the target cell by altering either the specific receptor site on the cell's outer surface or the virus's own envelope, to prevent the virus from fixing itself to the cell.

Anthony Fauci put it this way at the 1986 international meeting on AIDS that took place in Paris.

> It's unreasonable to assume that such an agent which exhibits all of these properties will become available within the reasonable future or ever. Therefore, investigators will of necessity have to accept certain compromises particularly in the area of manageable toxicity of drug and suppression, but not total elimination of the virus from the body. Although it seems unlikely that any anti-retroviral agent will be able to completely eliminate the virus and any remnant of viral genome [all the genetic information] from the host, one should expect that suppression of active viral replication is attainable. This could then set the stage for reconstitution of the immune system either spontaneously or therapeutically.

Against that background, and with the clear understanding that nothing yet has been wholly effective, here is a rundown of the most promising anti-AIDS drugs under investigation.

• Azidothymidine (AZT, also known as Compound S and BW A509U). The antiviral drug that has received the most media attention, AZT, which is obtained from herring sperm, was created in 1964 by Jerome Horowitz of the Michigan Cancer Foundation as a possible anticancer drug. Though it was unsuccessful, Burroughs Wellcome, the pharmaceutical company, tried it again, this time as an antibiotic. The attempt was also unsuccessful, and AZT wound up sitting on the lab shelf for some twenty years, waiting, as Dr. Samuel Broder, head of clinical oncology at the National Cancer Institute, put it, for a disease to come along.

When AIDS finally came along, AZT, it appeared, had some important features that might allow it to take advantage of the virus's peculiar method of reproducing. For one thing, AZT is actually an altered form of one of the natural chemical building blocks of the DNA molecule. It is believed now, after Broder's group used AZT successfully in 1985 against cultures of AIDS-infected human cells, that when the drug encounters the AIDS virus, it interferes with the way the virus replicates by forcing it to stop building its own DNA chain. It does this by replacing the real viral DNA — which the virus is making from RNA with its special enzyme — with AZT DNA. Essentially, the virus is tricked into inserting an incorrect molecule in the precisely orchestrated DNA chain, and because the error effectively blocks formation of viral DNA, it also stops the virus from multiplying. In effect, AZT forces the AIDS virus to commit suicide. AZT does not, however, affect the production of virus in cells already infected; it only prevents the virus from infecting new cells.

It wasn't long before AZT had progressed from the lab to "phase-I" clinical trials, the first potential AIDS drug to make that transition. (Phase-I trials involve giving an experimental drug to a small number of patients or normal volunteers to establish its pharmacokinetics and gather some initial safety information; phase-I trials of new anticancer drugs generally involve patients with the disease who have not responded to conventional treatment. In phase-II trials, the drug is given to more patients, at doses that have been determined safe in phase I, and both safety and efficacy are studied. More widespread administration of the drug comes during the controlled studies of phase III, while researchers try to determine the best dosages and learn more about adverse side effects.)

In March of 1986, after AZT tests had been run at the NCI, the University of Miami, and Duke University, the results were reported cautiously in *The Lancet* by Broder and seventeen other scientists. They gave the drug for 6 weeks to 11 patients with AIDS and to 8 who had ARC, and managed to get some improvement that had not resulted with any of the other previously tested drugs. Lab tests showed that the immune systems of 15 patients were working better; chronic fungus infections in 2 had cleared up without any other treatment; fever and night sweats quit in 6 others; in some instances, mouth ulcers lessened; and some cases of Kaposi's sarcoma regressed.

In a number of the patients who took the highest doses of AZT, cell cultures failed to turn up any trace of the AIDS virus. Moreover, the patients actually gained an average of five pounds apiece, a rather heartening response since AIDS victims generally waste away. The drug, also, could be given orally; side effects (some anemia and headaches) were not severe enough to stop the experiment; and fairly large amounts of the drug seemed to cross the blood-brain barrier. Apparently, AZT, unlike other treatments that try to control the symptoms of AIDS or boost the immune system, attacked the virus itself and also at least began to rearm the immune system.

By June of 1986, between 7 and 11 months after they started taking AZT, 16 of the original 19 were still alive, and most were still taking the drug. The longest survival time among those taking the drug has thus far been about 14 months.

Originally, those selected for the studies had to have either ARC or full-blown AIDS, which was defined for purposes of the study as one bout with *Pneumocystis carinii* pneumonia over 3 months (those with the pneumonia have died sooner, on the average, than those with Kaposi's sarcoma); their lab tests also had to fall within specific ranges to ensure that the patients were so matched that any benefits that occurred after AZT treatment were due to the drug itself and not to any individual peculiarities in the way the disease progresses.

Also, after 6 months on either AZT or placebos (neither the subjects nor the researchers were to know who was getting what), the trial was to be halted for a month and each patient tested further to measure results. If the pharmaceutical company determined that AZT was safe and effective, it was understood that all patients who participated would get the drug if they wanted it. The drug, however, was not plentiful, and although the manufacturer had said it had enough to treat more patients than are now treated, there was apparently not enough of it available to treat every AIDS patient under the so-called compassionate-use category set up by the FDA to allow doctors to prescribe an experimental drug for dying patients. (This is done at drug companies' discretion, since they must supply the drugs at cost or free of charge.)

The original rules raised a storm of protest — understandable after any success, no matter how modest, with a new drug against an untreatable, incurable disease. Hundreds of AIDS patients and their families called the manufacturer asking for the drug, and some even went in person to beg for it in the firm's lobby. Given the still-experimental nature of AZT, the dilemma was not to be easily resolved.

"It is not our charge to manufacture tons of material at great expense," observed microbiologist Dannie King, Burroughs Wellcome's AZT project director, "and jeopardize our other clinical programs, just to make sure everybody who wants it can have it. It is very, very expensive to make. I have to provide a stimulus to do this."[16] Simply put, that means firm evidence that AZT works, and is safe.

But in September 1986, the manufacturer announced that it was broadening the group eligible to receive AZT to include most of the 7,000 AIDS victims (of the 17,000 survivors of the disease at this writing) who were suffering from the pneumonia, and was dropping the placebo portion of the test. The reason: although there was still not enough firm evidence to talk about an AIDS cure, of 145 patients overall who had been given AZT, only 1 had died; of 137 who had received a placebo, 16 were dead. The drug was apparently prolonging lives. AZT would now be provided free of charge through physicians who agreed to share their research data. New criteria for eligibility were drawn up with almost unprecedented speed. These included:

- Documentation of one or more bouts with *Pneumo-cystis carinii* pneumonia.
- Not having received any previous drug therapy for AIDS.
- Not having received chemotherapy or other drugs that are toxic to the kidneys or bone marrow.
- Adequate liver and kidney function, and sufficiently high red- and white-blood-cell counts.
- Not being in any risk categories that include children,

pregnant women, and nursing mothers. (The criteria do not exclude patients with Kaposi's, so long as they are not receiving drug treatment. ARC patients are also now included.)

In March 1987, the FDA approved the use of AZT as a prescription drug against AIDS, emphasizing that it was not a cure. Distribution will still be limited to certain categories of patients because of the severe side effects — it can cause anemia serious enough to require frequent blood transfusions — and the short supply. But any doctor can prescribe it, at his or her discretion. (The cost of the drug is also quite high: $8,000 to $10,000 a year per patient.)

Researchers still have a way to go before they can make any blanket statements about the efficacy of AZT. They must, for instance, learn whether the short-term gains will persist, and whether the virus will develop a resistance to the drug. It may also work better when combined with alpha-interferon as some researchers have tried; and unquestioned safety must still be established. Moreover, researchers have to determine whether the immune shifts they observed were direct ones or were simply the result of the up-and-down course that AIDS so often runs through the bodies of its victims, or perhaps due to some placebo effect that raised spirits and increased appetites, thereby improving immune function. Sometimes merely taking part in a study of this kind can improve a person's health because the patient tends to get more medical attention than usual. (AIDS patients requiring information about AZT can call a toll-free number: 1-800-843-9388.)

• Dideoxycytidine (DDC). A sister compound of AZT, this drug has been shown to block replication of the AIDS and other retroviruses in laboratory cultures. Manufactured by Hoffmann–La Roche, it has also been effective when given orally in tests with dogs. Some researchers initially suspected that DDC would prove to be at least as effective as AZT, and less toxic. But although early lab tests seemed to confirm those beliefs, the first human trials have found the drug to be highly toxic. Researchers are looking into the effects of lower dosages.

• CS-85. Developed by scientists at Emory University, the Veterans Administration Medical Center, and the University of Georgia, this drug appears to inhibit the growth of the AIDS virus at a level comparable to AZT. It has the additional advantage of being at least ten times less toxic to human bone marrow cells than AZT. When it was added to human cells that had been mixed with the AIDS virus, the drug specifically targeted the infected cells and stopped, almost completely, the replication of the virus — a sign that the virus would not spread to other, uninfected cells.

According to Dr. Raymond F. Schinazi, a viral pharmacologist at Emory, the next step is to determine exactly how the drug works. Although its chemical structure is similar to that of AZT, the action of CS-85 appears to be different from AZT's and perhaps involves intervention at a later stage in the replication cycle of the AIDS virus.

• Glycyrrhizin. A component of licorice, this substance has been used to treat hepatitis and various allergies, and reportedly is capable of stimulating the immune system as well. According to Japanese scientists, who have been testing it in the laboratory, it has proven effective in halting growth of the AIDS virus. When researchers at Fukushima Medical College and the Yamaguchi University Medical School recently bathed AIDS-infected lymphocytes with the chemical, they found that some 80 percent survived; by contrast, most of the virus-infected cells that were not treated with the chemical died within three days. Moreover, when the glycyrrhizin solution was doubled in density, the survival rate among the infected lymphocytes was almost identical to that of cells that were not infected with the AIDS virus at all. Thus far, no clinical trials have been conducted.

• Anti-gene. This is not a drug therapy, nor is it even, at the moment, any form of therapy. Anti-gene is, however, an intriguing, wholly experimental way of inhibiting AIDS-virus replication — one that works, as does AZT, by blocking the copying function in the virus's genetic material and thus disrupting the orderly instructions for making new viruses. Thus far it has been tested only in laboratory flasks and dishes — on cultures of human white blood cells infected with the AIDS virus — but it could eventually have some therapeutic value. The new approach, which has drawn little if any media attention, was reported on in June of 1986 in the *Proceedings of the National Academy of Sciences* by Paul Zamecnik of the Worcester (Massachusetts) Foundation for Experimental Biology, a scientist widely regarded as a pioneer in protein biosynthesis and genetic-coding mechanisms.

Zamecnik's experiment involves synthesizing, by chemical means, a short piece of DNA that binds precisely to a critical portion of the AIDS virus's genetic material — the part that contains specific template instructions for making new virus. The foundation's scientific director, Dr. Thoru Pederson, used the following analogy to describe the process:

Consider a newspaper printing press. If all the type set for the page's right-hand column was selectively covered, letter by letter, with little metal caps before running the press, the resulting printed pages would be incomplete and therefore, from a journalistic perspective, nonfunctional. In Dr. Zamecnik's work, a short piece of DNA is similarly used to specifically fit over a segment of code letters in the AIDS virus's genetic blueprint.[17]

When Zamecnik's anti-gene was tested on blood cells, the results were startling: it inhibited AIDS-virus replication and gene expression by 80 percent to 95 percent. Of special note also was the finding that not all sections of the virus's genetic material are equally susceptible to the anti-gene. There were, instead, preferred targets for blocking — an especially significant finding in that it will, it is hoped, enable researchers to design even more efficient anti-genes.

Zamecnik's work with the AIDS virus actually grew out of experiments he did eight years earlier. Then, he synthesized a small piece of DNA that fit exactly, lock-and-key fashion, onto a vital portion of the genetic material of a virus that causes cancer in rodents. When cells harboring this virus were treated with the anti-gene, replication of the virus was blocked.

Next, Zamecnik will focus on whether the method can be

applied to the whole body. To that end, he and his colleagues are trying to modify the anti-gene chemically to make it more resistant to inactivation in the bloodstream. Conceivably, the anti-gene could be delivered intravenously in the form of liposomes, microscopic fatty capsules that already have been used to carry potent antifungal drugs into the bodies of cancer patients in order to treat life-threatening infections.

• Ribavirin. Used against flu in seventy countries and active against RNA viruses as well as DNA viruses, this drug (marketed under the name Virazole by ICN Pharmaceuticals) was synthesized by Roland Robins of the Nucleic Acid Research Institute and Joseph T. Witkowski some years ago. In January of 1986, the FDA approved its use only in aerosol form to treat severe infections caused by the respiratory syncytial virus (RSV), an especially nasty agent that kills some 5,000 infants a year and hospitalizes 100,000. (Many AIDS and ARC patients have been able to obtain the drug in Mexico and have been self-administering it.)

According to Dr. Robins, ribavirin has been studied in more animals and against more viruses than any other antiviral agent, and is active in cell culture against 85 percent of all viruses studied, including a leukemia virus in animals. (The drug appears to have no effect, however, against the polio virus, certain coxsackieviruses, pseudorabies virus, and hepatitis B.) Moreover, says Robins, its broad-spectrum antiviral activity is greater than that of any other such known agent, including interferon.[18]

In various laboratory studies, ribavirin has been found to inhibit replication of the AIDS virus with a minimum amount of damage to the infected cells, and to increase the number of T-4 cells. Preliminary clinical trials are currently under way on a small number of patients, and eight others aimed at treating pre-AIDS patients are planned. In one earlier trial in New York, 27 gay men with AIDS-virus infection but without symptoms received the drug orally; reverse-transcriptase activity in cultures of blood lymphocytes decreased but was not eliminated. There were also dose-related side effects, among them anemia, nausea, headache, fatigue, and labored breathing on exertion. (Recently, scientists at Massachusetts General Hospital discovered that when ribavirin and AZT are mixed in a test tube, they are "antagonistic" — that is, they cancel each other out. Theoretically, if AIDS patients take both drugs — as they might if they buy black-market supplies — the efficacy of either, probably more so AZT, would be weakened.)

• Foscarnet (trisodium phosphonoformate, also called PFA). This powerful drug (made by Astra in Sweden), which can inhibit reverse transcriptase, is active against several herpes viruses (which often cause severe secondary infections in AIDS patients). In the laboratory, it has blocked replication of the AIDS virus. Several phase-I clinical trials are under way in the United States, Sweden, and Denmark. But there are several drawbacks. One is that the drug must be given intravenously, which rules out long-term therapy. When continuous infusions of Foscarnet were given to 3 AIDS patients at the NIH recently, acute kidney failure developed in all of them, and the trial was discontinued. (That trial has since been redesigned with lower doses.) Apart from its potentially dangerous effect on the kidneys, Foscarnet is also retained for long periods in bone tissue. For these reasons, it is doubtful the drug will ever be widely used in AIDS.

• HPA-23 (antimoniotungstate). The mineral compound (made by Rhone-Poulenc of France) used in Paris to treat actor Rock Hudson, this is another drug that inhibits reverse transcriptase. It does not rid the body of the virus, but only keeps it from multiplying and spreading to other cells. Some 200 patients have been treated with HPA-23 in France, but although it reduced or cleared the AIDS virus from the blood in some cases, there have been no long-term benefits, and viral activity returned after the drug was discontinued. Made from two heavy metals, antimony and tungsten, the drug causes liver dysfunction and, since it is toxic to blood platelets (the blood-clotting cells), bleeding.

Clinical trials are now under way, but it is still much too early to tell whether the drug is safe and effective. At the 1986 Paris AIDS meeting, HPA-23 was cited as an agent that has not lived up to its early reputation. "Investigators are not impressed that it's prolonged any lives," said virologist Martin S. Hirsch of the

Massachusetts General Hospital. "Even though a large number
of patients have been treated with it, we still don't know if it
has any real benefit because there have been no controlled
trials."

• AL-721. An antiviral compound developed by Praxis Pharmaceuticals, this agent, which has been used to treat the symptoms of drug withdrawal, seems to interfere with the receptor
process whereby the AIDS virus attaches to and infects host
cells, disrupting both the key and the lock required for infection.
According to the company, it readily penetrates the brain, one
of the critical target sites for the virus. In July 1986, Dr. Arnold
Lippa, the firm's president, informed a congressional subcommittee reviewing issues dealing with the development of AIDS
drugs that phase-I clinical trials with AL-721 had been com-
pleted in normal volunteers; there were no toxic effects at doses
800-percent higher than the anticipated therapeutic doses. At
this writing, phase-II trials designed to test the drug's efficacy
in patients with ARC were under way at St. Luke's–Roosevelt
Hospital in New York City, and in London.

• Ansamycin (LM-427). Used to treat some of the opportunistic
infections associated with AIDS (primarily *Mycobacterium avium
intracellulare*), this drug (made by Farmitalia of Italy) seems to
also have some effect against the virus itself. Laboratory studies
are continuing.

• DHPG. This drug has a jaw-breaking chemical name: 9-(1,3-
Dihydroxy-2-propoxymethyl)guanine. Like ansamycin, it is now
being tried primarily as a treatment for an opportunistic infection of AIDS, one caused by the cytomegalovirus (CMV). As
was noted earlier, the CMV virus infects virtually everyone at
some time in his or her life, and it usually causes a mild infection,
except when it strikes those with weak immune systems. When
it does that, it can be quite dangerous. The infections it causes
are, in fact, one of the primary causes of death in AIDS patients.
CMV infection has been untreatable, but DHPG seems able to
control it in certain patients temporarily.

In a recent study involving researchers across the country, 26
extremely sick patients thought to be dying from CMV infection
were given DHPG on a compassionate-use basis. Twenty-two

of them had AIDS, 2 had received bone marrow transplants, 1 had a congenital immunodeficiency disease, and 1 was receiving immunosuppressive drugs. Although all were believed to have CMV infection when they first got the drug, the researchers determined later that 4 probably did not. Among the remaining 22, 17 showed some clinical improvement; 5 died before completion of the fourteen-day experiment, without any apparent benefit. Unfortunately, despite the initial improvement, most of the patients eventually had relapses, and a majority died within ten months of treatment. Nonetheless, the researchers were encouraged.

"This is certainly not a cure for AIDS and not even a cure for CMV," said Dr. Thomas Merigan of Stanford University School of Medicine, the chairman of the study group.

> But it is a foot in the door in a situation where we really had no effective treatment approach before. The important thing is that we can reproducibly suppress CMV infection with this drug. It's the only way we've got right now to get this virus. However, with a disease like AIDS, you have such profound immune suppression that the moment you stop treating with the drug, the infection recurs. Among the patients who were helped, as long as they kept getting the drug, the disease was held back. Therefore, we're looking for ways to give it safely for long periods of time, or to combine it with other treatments to get enduring suppression of CMV.[19]

• Eflornithine hydrochloride. Newly developed (by Dow Chemical), this drug has gotten good marks in early tests as a treatment for *Pneumocystis carinii,* the form of pneumonia so often fatal to AIDS patients. The drug has been tried in 150 patients who had not responded to other forms of treatment; of 66 on whom data were obtained, three-quarters were cured of the pneumonia. Tests are still under way.

• Suramin. Widely used to treat African trypanosomiasis (sleeping sickness) and onchocerciasis (a disease caused by a worm parasite), this drug is a prime example of early research enthusiasm giving way to disappointment. When the drug — another reverse-transcriptase inhibitor — was first tried on a handful of patients at the NIH, it seemed to clear the AIDS virus from the blood of several of them. But there was no clinical or immunologic improvement, and the virus returned when the drug treatment was stopped. Longer-term studies with a few more patients have given researchers pause about the safety as well as the efficacy of suramin. It now not only does not appear to suppress the virus substantially, but is quite toxic, causing urinary and liver difficulties, fever, rashes, and burning sensations in the extremities.

"In addition, and most importantly," Anthony Fauci told the 1986 Paris AIDS meeting, "several patients appeared to worsen clinically on the drug, particularly with acceleration of Kaposi's sarcoma. Clearly, suramin should not be used as a single agent in the treatment of AIDS. The experience with it strongly underscores the need for long-range controlled clinical studies before any drug is made widely available for the treatment of AIDS, even those drugs which may show some suggestion of laboratory benefit in limited short-range studies."

• Peptide T. This potential anti-AIDS drug may work by preventing the virus from entering cells. Swedish investigators at the Karolinska Institute administered the drug to 4 severely ill AIDS patients in late 1986 on a compassionate-use basis and found that it seemed to alleviate their symptoms without any ill effects. When the drug was withdrawn, the men's conditions worsened, promoting the Swedish government to grant permission to the Karolinska scientists to administer the drug again for six months. At the same time, the researchers will begin testing peptide T against a placebo in 36 AIDS patients; phase-I studies are under way.

It is perhaps appropriate to comment here on two related issues that have generally been overlooked amid all the discussion of drug development and testing: whether the use of a placebo in drug trials for so lethal a disease as AIDS is correct, and whether every AIDS patient who wants an experimental drug should get it, even though it has not been put through long-term studies. There is a good deal of agonizing over these questions.

AIDS patients who feel they have nothing to lose by taking an experimental drug, even one that might make them worse, argue that it is unfair and immoral to deny them such medication on demand, even if they are enrolled in a double-blind, placebo-controlled, randomized clinical trial in which they have a fifty-fifty chance of getting the drug or a sugar pill (no one knows which, not the patient or the researcher who is conducting the study). Here is how one AIDS patient participating in the original AZT trial (before the drug was released for wider consumption) expressed his frustration:

It's an absolute mind-blower. It's true guinea pig city. They're rather arrogant. They know they've got you, because they're holding out this thread of a chance of life. For the first month you have to travel to the hospital at your own expense once a week for blood tests and other exams. Now it's every other week. And it's supposed to be the same day of the week each time. You can only be one day late. They give you just enough capsules, maybe a couple extra, to keep you going until your next appointment. You have to take them every four hours, even during the night, and you're not supposed to take them within an hour of eating. That's the hardest part, planning your meals, because AIDS does strange things to your appetite. And then you realize you're going through all this agony and you might be bringing home sugar pills.

I had a real shock one week when I casually mentioned that I had taken aspirin. They practically went into orbit. They want you cold turkey on everything. I sure as hell could use some tranquilizers, I'm so distraught over this disease. I have taken some drugs to control other things, but I haven't told them. I don't tell them all my symptoms, either. This is life and death we're talking about here. The word is that once you're on the study they really don't want to throw you off because they don't want to lose a patient, lose that data. But who wants to take a chance?

I assume all the blood they draw is sent away [he's never told how he's doing, and he doesn't ask], and they don't even know the results themselves because it might bias them. And if they did know everything, I assume they wouldn't tell. But I'm having tests run, trying to monitor it on my own. The other thing I'd like to do is take the capsules to a lab and have them analyzed to see if they're placebos, but I haven't gotten very far with that. I asked the doctor about it and he was offended. I'd probably keep going through the motions so as not to hurt my chances of ever getting the drug. And I might try to get into another drug program. But I'd have to lie and sneak around to do that because they wouldn't want somebody who was already in the AZT study. And anyway, there aren't any other drugs that have shown any promise, are there? I went to Mexico to get ribavirin, and that didn't do me any good. I wish I were getting this drug, I really do. They told me that if I was on the placebo there's no guarantee I'll ever get the drug. I'll be first on the list to get it, if they decide it works. But God knows when they'll have the results. And time is such a factor in this disease.[20]

Researchers say that such an attitude is fairly common — and understandable — among patients who find that a placebo-controlled study is their only chance to try a drug that might help. On the other hand, they argue, while any drug test ideally should benefit both the subjects and future patients, it just does not work that way all the time, for there is simply no way other than giving placebos to some AIDS patients and the real drug to the rest to establish a drug's effectiveness conclusively.

Moreover, the scientists maintain, turning an experimental drug loose for everyone who wants it, instead of confining it to small groups of subjects, as the AIDS drugs are, would be ethically undesirable even if a company had enormous quantities in stock. Not only would it be impossible to run a placebo-controlled test — since an AIDS patient would be able to get the drug easily and would hardly want to enter a trial that gave him only a fifty-fifty chance of receiving it — but an unproven, possibly worthless, and perhaps dangerous drug would come into widespread use.

But besides altruism, there is the financial consideration: millions of dollars to develop large quantities of a drug that may not work, and to combat a disease that probably never will become a threat to the vast majority of people. Burroughs Wellcome is paying the entire $5-million cost of the AZT trial, a system of financing drug research that is, as one AIDS specialist puts it, "like asking private industry to do the Manhattan Project."[21]

AN AIDS VACCINE?

Talk about vaccines and chances are no one will mention Edward Jenner, who gave us the name, as well as a way to protect humankind against smallpox. Nor Almroth Edward Wright, who developed a typhoid vaccine; or Waldemar Haffkine and his two vaccines against cholera. But the names of Sabin and Salk come readily to mind, perhaps because they had the advantage of working in the glare of media publicity, and because it was not so long ago that polio hysteria, not unlike that associated with AIDS, was sweeping the country. Jonas Salk's injectable, killed-virus vaccine was greeted with a worldwide sense of relief when it was licensed in 1955; seven years later, Albert Sabin's name showed up in Sabin Oral Sundays (SOS), and the weakened-virus vaccine he developed, in sugar cubes.

When and if an AIDS vaccine is developed, the scientist or scientists whose names are associated with it will, given the emphasis today's electronic media place on research breakthroughs, undoubtedly achieve a notoriety at least equal to that associated with Salk and Sabin — if it does not eclipse it.

But will AIDS produce, as polio did, a Salk or a Sabin? It is possible, but the event is certainly not just around the corner. Sabin himself, now eighty and working as an NIH consultant in a basement room in Bethesda, is dubious. When I approached him recently to ask what he thought about the prospects of someone developing an AIDS vaccine, his answer, though delivered slowly, between bites of a tuna salad sandwich, was not a hedge:

> Many people, including some of my colleagues, think in simplistic terms. You have an infectious disease, you make a vaccine that'll make antibodies against it, and bingo! But that's not the way it works in polio, and not quite the way it works in measles. You have to understand the nature

of the disease. In measles, one infection will produce life-long immunity. But with AIDS, the production of anti-bodies isn't enough. The person acquires the infection, then develops an immunity as measured by the antibodies, but then continues to carry the virus in certain blood cells and can still transmit the disease. The fact that people who develop some immune manifestations aren't protected against further progress of the disease speaks against making a vaccine. But we have to try.

Which is what dozens of researchers are doing in a few laboratories here and abroad. An AIDS vaccine developed by Dr. Salk may, indeed, be lab-tested shortly. But unlike their counterparts who are regularly testing drugs on AIDS patients, most vaccine hunters are not yet ready for wide-scale human trials.

In March of 1987, Daniel Zagury of the Pierre and Marie Curie University in Paris made headlines by injecting himself with a potential vaccine, while his colleagues tried it on several patients in Africa. And the following August, federal officials announced plans for the first human trials in this country of an experimental AIDS vaccine — while warning at the same time that its use as an effective preventive, like that of any other vaccine, was still many years away. But for the most part, the best that vaccine researchers have been able to do thus far is to test, in the laboratory and in some animals, a variety of likely protein antigens from the AIDS virus that have been meticulously identified, extracted, altered, and reproduced, by a bewildering array of techniques that would have spun even the heads of Salk and Sabin back in the fifties, not to mention that of Edward Jenner.

A few of these proteins have stimulated the antibodies — which, theoretically at least, would prevent a case of the disease from showing up. How effective they will be if made into an actual vaccine remains to be seen. "We must be clever in the way we make vaccines," Harvard's William Haseltine warned scientists at the 1986 Paris AIDS meeting. "When you listen to the vaccine data at this meeting and at future meetings, ask yourself, 'Have these vaccine preparations done any better than the virus itself?' "

Haseltine was referring to something pointed to earlier in this book: that while people infected with the AIDS virus generally produce antibodies, those natural antibodies offer no protection against the virus; some antibodies, present in greater numbers, also recognize certain proteins in the core of the virus that are not implicated in the infection process and these antibodies have no protective capability. Thus, a vaccine that simply stimulates antibodies artificially may well be just as ineffective, unless, as Haseltine put it, the scientists are more clever than the virus.

So far, the mindless virus, an agent that may not even be "alive" in the classic sense, is ahead. Trying to come up with an AIDS vaccine, scientists are painfully aware, is not the same as developing one against other viruses, even though the basic strategy and the mechanism of action are virtually the same: first, obtain a virus from a human carrier's blood, or from an infected animal or cultured cells; if the whole virus is used, disable it just enough so it does not cause disease but produces antibodies against it, and inoculate someone with it; the person's immune system records that first encounter as it puts out specific antibodies to the foreign antigens, and, whenever the real thing gets into the body — even many years later — the primed immune cells, bearing the indelible "mark" of the intruder, remember the original onslaught, and attack it. It can all be quite neatly described textbook-fashion, but, as Sabin and Haseltine have suggested, with AIDS, an especially lethal virus that does not always behave by the rules that have governed the production of other vaccines, it is not that simple.

Apart from the fact that the antibodies produced against an AIDS-virus infection do not seem to be doing the patient much good, one has to consider that most of the vaccines currently in use are made from live viruses that have been sufficiently weakened so that they no longer cause the disease yet stimulate people who are vaccinated into producing their own antibodies. (The Salk vaccine uses a polio virus that is first grown outside the body, then destroyed and injected to produce antibodies. The problem with it is that it requires periodic booster shots and must be given to everyone who needs protection. The weakened virus used in the Sabin vaccine, on the other hand, requires no booster, provides lifelong immunity, and also protects those who have not taken it because it is excreted from the body, exposing others to it, and, thus, protects those who are merely in contact with it.)

But with a virus as dangerous as the one that causes AIDS, using a live virus that has been weakened in the conventional way is playing with a biological time bomb, for it is possible that it could somehow regain strength and reactivate itself. (Even with the attenuated Sabin vaccine, it has been suggested, a case of polio will result in one in a million doses.) Certain forms of the AIDS virus, also, have known cancer-causing activity, and an attenuated-virus vaccine might carry a residue of gene products that could promote the development of a malignancy. Another drawback is the AIDS virus's ability to change its antigen (protein) coat; researchers note extensive diversity in the genetic structure of different isolates of the AIDS virus, especially in the envelope genes, the ones that produce the proteins in the virus's coat, and many of these strains can cause AIDS.

These viral proteins are the critical ones that trigger neutralizing antibodies in infected individuals; thus, the many variations seen in the envelope mean that antibodies summoned up against one variant of the AIDS virus may be worthless against a possible wide range of others. (Such shifting is not, as we have seen, an uncommon occurrence with viruses, which often undergo an "antigenic drift," changing sufficiently so as to render ineffective any vaccine that has been successful, for a time, against them. Polio, for example, has but 3 viral variations; the common cold, 115.) However, Daniel Zagury found that when he put samples of his immune cells after vaccination in a test tube and added two very different strains of AIDS virus, more immune cells grew in response to the challenge. This effect is heartening, since it suggests that a vaccine may, indeed, protect against a variety of AIDS strains.

Even with the persistent mutations that characterize the AIDS virus, hope for a vaccine is still fairly high. Part of the guarded optimism is inspired by the recently approved hepatitis-B vaccine, which employs a genetic-engineering approach that may be (and indeed, would have to be) applied to the development of an AIDS vaccine. Its development — which does not rely, as did the previous version, on blood from people already infected with the disease but on a gene from the hepatitis virus — has already been hailed by FDA commissioner Frank Young as one that "opens a new era in vaccine production, one that opens the door for the production of other vaccines that have so far been impractical, potentially unsafe or impossible to make."[22]

The new vaccine was developed by the Chiron Corporation of Emeryville, California, and scientists at the University of California at San Francisco and the University of Washington. Merck Sharp & Dohme, which also makes and markets the older hepatitis vaccine, is selling the new one under the name Recombivax HB. Its development is truly remarkable, not only from a technical standpoint, but because there is still no treatment and no cure for the disease it prevents, one that is carried by more than 200 million people worldwide.

It also circumvents the consumer problems that had developed over the earlier vaccine. Because antibodies form not in response to the entire virus but to the antigen in the protein coat that surrounds the virus, vaccine makers must, of course, zero in on that portion. But they generally use the whole virus in the process. Although the first vaccine, made from a carrier's blood, was proved safe and effective, fears were raised that it could contain not only inactivated hepatitis organisms but the AIDS virus since many of those who had hepatitis and who donated the plasma to make the vaccine were homosexuals or IV-drug abusers.

Despite studies demonstrating that the heat and chemical treatments used to purify the vaccine remove or inactivate any AIDS virus that might be present, and that people who receive the vaccine do not get AIDS that way, fear of AIDS, nevertheless, helped limit acceptance of the existing vaccine. Enter the new, genetically engineered product, which uses only the antigen and not the whole virus — a process that makes the vaccine, unlike other vaccines, incapable of generating the disease it is designed to prevent. Here is how the scientists prepared what is now known as a subunit vaccine:

The gene that directs production of the surface antigen is removed from the virus and spliced into common intestinal bacteria. The bacteria, in turn, produce quantities of DNA containing the surface antigen gene. The DNA, which codes for the surface antigen gene, is removed and purified, then transplanted into yeast cells, which produce large quantities of the surface antigen as they grow. The surface antigen is removed, concentrated, and purified. The last step involves adding chemicals to increase potency, and preservatives, and testing to assure sterility and purity.

Before it all got off the ground, however, the researchers had to take a few enormously important steps, not the least of which was determining which specific genes were most likely responsible for making the surface antigen of the virus, and for the location and structure of the crucial antigen sites.

Because antibodies to the AIDS virus are indeed generated, albeit weakly, it obviously follows that antigens on or in the virus provoke them. Finding those antigens, theoretically, means that a subunit vaccine using only simulated or identical parts of the deadly virus could be made to work safely.

One bright ray in that direction came when scientists in Max Essex's laboratory at Harvard discovered that the simian AIDS virus, STLV-III, seems to have some surface antigens that are not only very similar to those of the human AIDS virus, but are also surprisingly stable over time. This indicated that although the AIDS virus has a lot of variability in its envelope genes, there appear to be areas in the coat that are "conserved" — that is, there are identical portions among different strains that do not show antigenic drift, or mutation.

Subsequent antibody testing has shown that specific glycoproteins (compounds made up of a protein and a carbohydrate) in the virus's envelope do provoke immune responses in mice, guinea pigs, rabbits, and rhesus monkeys. Because these substances seem to be the main targets of antibodies produced by the body as an immune response to the virus, they have become the focus of the vaccine hunters. (In order to make the glycoproteins more visible to the immune system's cells, and to provoke the most vigorous response, researchers use artificial-membrane matrices, called ISCOM — for "immune-stimulating complexes" — to anchor the viral subunits they are testing.)

Most of the research, aimed at determining not only whether these subunits stimulate antibodies but whether the reaction is a protective one as well, has concentrated on an antibody-stimulator called gp120, the largest protein on the AIDS-virus envelope, and among the ones that do not change. (Essex has found that gp120 and gp160 are the major target antigens for antibodies from patients with AIDS and ARC, and from some healthy homosexual men.) Gp120 appears to be a promising choice. Animals, for example, can be given the protein that has been produced conventionally (that is, by extracting it from live AIDS virus taken from carriers and then grown in tissue culture), and, when the antibodies it produces are, in turn, put into culture dishes, the antibodies seem to prevent the destruction of the cells when the AIDS virus is introduced. The technique has also induced a protective response in preliminary tests with goats and rhesus monkeys.

But even more exciting, and far safer, is a recombinant-derived version of gp120 that has been used for the first time to produce antibodies that protect human cells in tissue culture from infection by the AIDS virus. Produced only recently by Genentech, the San Francisco–based gene-engineering firm, gp120 is made by inserting the gene that codes for it into mammalian cells (from hamster ovaries), which then churn out quantities of the protein that mimics the one that naturally encases the AIDS virus. Although a gp120-like molecule had been synthesized by several laboratories in yeast and bacteria cells, these systems, according to Genentech, do not have the capability that mammalian cells have to process the correct antigenic structure necessary to produce strongly neutralizing antibodies.

Moreover, use of the mammalian culture system may prove to be highly efficient if gp120 ever gets to commercial production, since it enables much more material to be produced: scientists say they are able to get the same yield of gp120 protein in 1 liter of mammalian culture that would require approximately 400 liters of AIDS-virus culture. (At the present time, it takes around 60 gallons of tissue culture to grow a pint of pure AIDS virus, from which gp120 is extracted.)

The next step is to evaluate gp120 antibody response in primates sensitive to the human AIDS virus, notably chimpanzees, by injecting the animals with the vaccine prototype, then challenging them with the virus to see if it really protects against infection. (This, incidentally, is not always easy to do, since chimps are in incredibly short supply, and keepers get a $20,000-a-year user fee.)

There is, of course, the possibility that primates, including the highest of that order, man, will respond differently from rodents and every other living thing that gp120 is tried on, and may not demonstrate the same neutralizing antibody reply simply because immune systems do vary. Merely building envelope proteins that look like the real thing does not mean that effective immunity will follow. As Haseltine has argued, although the ability of the anti-gp120 antibodies to bind to the AIDS virus seems to be strong, their power to neutralize the AIDS virus, to stop it from replicating, is relatively weak. Scientists know that antibodies may be able to stop free viruses in their tracks, and thus prevent them from infecting a new cell; but getting at the virus once it has already infected a cell, and is on its way to fusing with a nearby healthy cell so it can replicate, is quite another matter. When the AIDS virus spreads this way, it is not exactly a clear target. On the other hand, scientists think that the key to protecting someone against AIDS lies in producing the antibodies *before* exposure to the virus occurs, which is, of course, what a vaccine is all about.

Several other approaches besides using gp120 are being tried. One that has aroused considerable interest circumvents the ability of the AIDS virus to change the color of its coat, so to speak. Perhaps, researchers reason, by zeroing in on the virus's core proteins, which may not change as frequently as the envelope while the virus replicates, a better, more stable, target for a vaccine may be found. The core proteins go by the simple scientific nickname gag; and, according to some new research by Allan Goldstein of George Washington University and scientists at the National Cancer Institute, these core proteins are remarkably similar to thymosin, the human hormone mentioned earlier, in the discussion of biological-response modifiers. That similarity, Goldstein believes, may be the AIDS virus's Achilles' heel.

Usually, levels of thymosin, which helps to regulate T-cells, are way down in patients suffering from immune deficiency diseases. But surprisingly, and somewhat paradoxically, levels of the hormone seem to be *elevated* in many AIDS patients — apparently, it now turns out, as the result of the virus's supply of thymosin look-alike in its core. To see where the similarity between the two forms of thymosin might lead, Goldstein and his colleagues created a synthetic version of the hormone and injected it into rabbits, which eventually produced antibodies to it. The next step was to determine whether the antibodies would attack the real thymosin in the virus's core. Using the antibodies, the scientists prepared a serum that reacted with the synthetic thymosin; when they tested it against infected human cells in test tubes, the serum markedly reduced levels of the core protein and, thus, prevented the AIDS virus from replicating in the cells; the serum also hampered production of the virus's reverse transcriptase.

Goldstein believes that an effective AIDS vaccine could be made either from the synthetic thymosin or from the protein produced by the virus's gag gene. But, as in virtually all potentially useful medicines, there is a tradeoff. The very similarity between the naturally produced hormone and the stuff in the virus's core that provides a clue to an AIDS vaccine could pose a problem: antibodies produced against the protein could fail to tell the difference between the two, and thus might cause the body to attack its own thymus, where the real thymosin, as well as T-cells, are produced. This phenomenon may, in fact, explain why AIDS victims, who often have severely damaged thymus glands, cannot seem to fight off the disease. Any antibodies made against the viral protein simply may not recognize the thymus as "self," might, in effect, regard it as the virus, and attack it as well, thereby preventing the T-cells from doing their job. Primate studies, now under way, may provide an answer soon, and if the approach works the way it is supposed to, it could serve as the basis for a vaccine that would be produced by Viral Technologies, Inc., a Washington, D.C., biomedical company that is the keeper of the technique's proprietary technology.

Both thymosin and AZT employ trickery to achieve their

objectives: antibodies are made to go after thymosin in the virus as well as in a synthetic state; and in the AZT approach, the virus is fooled into inserting an incorrect, altered form of DNA into its own growing chain. Another example of laboratory trickery employed to take advantage of the sometime gullibility of a microorganism fools certain immune-system cells into making antibodies against an invader disguised as the AIDS virus, then uses them to ward off the real culprit if it shows up. In this case, the invader is the vaccinia virus, the cowpox-causing agent that was the basis for Edward Jenner's smallpox vaccine, far and away the most widely used vaccine ever developed against a human disease. Two U.S. research teams — from the National Institute of Allergy and Infectious Diseases, and Oncogen, a Bristol-Myers subsidiary in Seattle — recently remodeled the vaccinia virus by inserting a key gene from the AIDS virus (the envelope gene that codes for gp120) into it. When the rebuilt virus, now producing AIDS-virus surface proteins, was injected into mice and monkeys, and also mixed with cultured cells, antibodies against its new coat were produced, indicating that the virus was being treated as a real AIDS virus.

Later, researchers were able to elicit a second type of immune response, known as cell-mediated immunity. This is the other defense mechanism essential to warding off a virus attack. While merely producing antibodies does not necessarily mean they will protect the body, the induction of cell-mediated immunity is a bit more promising since it depends on the coordinated activity of the helper T-cells and the killer T-cells. When scientists injected the genetically engineered experimental vaccine into monkeys, then exposed their blood to purified AIDS virus, not only were antibodies produced, but so, too, were activated T-cells that proliferated and produced defender interleukin-2. Monkeys who were then given booster doses of the vaccine followed the same pattern: they developed antibodies, activated T-cells, and interleukin-2. Chimps were also inoculated with the vaccine, and they, too, produced both helper and killer T-cells. Theoretically, if those antibodies were given as a vaccine, they would be primed to attack the surface molecules of an actual AIDS virus should it enter someone's body.

Vaccinia's advantage is that it is relatively safe — although in rare instances it has some dangerous side effects, particularly if it is given to someone with immune defenses compromised by AIDS. Because of that potential, some researchers feel that the celebrated vaccine should not be taken out of storage unless some deadly disease suddenly becomes the serious global threat that smallpox was. Thus far, nothing about AIDS justifies that characterization — which is not to say that using vaccinia in an AIDS vaccine is unwarranted. If it works in immunizing against AIDS, it may not be any more dangerous than it was when it was used against smallpox, its rare side effects notwithstanding.

Scientists are not as certain, however, about what some are calling the vaccine of last resort. This one would take the somewhat risky tack of using the entire AIDS virus itself, but either with its tat gene (the one that it needs to grow) cut out by genetic surgery, or with the virus altered enough so that it does not kill T-cells. With the tat gene removed, a feat announced simultaneously in 1986 by Haseltine and Flossie Wong-Staal of the NCI, the virus does not kill T-cells, and because it cannot reproduce, it is, for all intents and purposes, dead. Because it has the same antigens as the original virus, it would look the same to the immune system and, thus, would trigger an immunogenic response.

A few months after the tat work was announced, NCI scientists revealed they had created another version of a mutant AIDS virus by cutting out five amino acids from an envelope gene. The altered virus is still infectious, still goes after T-cells, and still replicates with but a piece of its gene removed; but what is important is that it does not seem to kill T-cells. Theoretically, the altered viruses could be the basis for an AIDS vaccine, and would be far safer than one derived from the wild, or natural, virus.

There is also potential in these experiments for an antiviral attack that could help in treatment of those already infected with AIDS. If, for example, the altered virus is given to an AIDS patient, it might compete with the wild virus for space in cells still uninfected; eventually it could win out, crowding out the wild virus, protecting cells from future infection, and helping to preserve some immune function. "Hopefully, you would always preserve a population of target cells," said Wong-Staal. "The ones infected by the wild virus will die, but the others will be protected. You won't completely deplete the pool."[23] Again, there is the uncertainty about the safety of using an intact, even an altered virus, as a vaccine or in treatment. Researchers still do not know if these essentially disarmed agents are capable of finding new ways to infect cells, grow in an entirely new range of cells, or wreak some yet unknown havoc throughout the body.

Finally, as with the various experimental AIDS drugs, developing, testing, approving, and eventually marketing an AIDS vaccine raises a number of other important issues besides the critical question of whether a vaccine would even be an effective barrier in a peculiar disease like AIDS, or would offer any protection against the many variants of the virus. First of all, there is the possibility that some members of high-risk groups would feel a vaccine gives them carte blanche to resume dangerous practices. Given the unlikelihood that an AIDS vaccine would be 100-percent effective — and also the fact that it would not be a barrier against other sexually transmitted diseases, or against needle-borne hepatitis — some of those at high risk could remain so.

In addition, there are the enormous costs, an estimated $10 million to $30 million to develop a vaccine, and maybe another $20 million for clinical trials. Also, many drug firms are reluctant to get into the vaccine-development business because of the fear of lawsuits that might arise if a rash of side effects breaks out when the drug is tested or marketed. The whooping-cough vaccine is a case in point: it has been the object of a flood of lawsuits stemming from allegations that it causes neurological defects and sudden infant death. (Many of the alleged injuries, it turns out, have not been found to be vaccine-caused.) To get around the threat of litigation, several genetic-engineering firms are seeking passage of legislation (notably in California, where Genentech and Chiron are located) that would limit the liability of manufacturers of an AIDS vaccine, and also sweeten the research pot by providing incentives.

Such efforts to speed up development of an AIDS vaccine do, of course, make sense. As Stanford University infectious-diseases specialist Thomas C. Merigan puts it:

> Spreading the cost of risk throughout the society is the best approach to deal with vaccines because we will never have an absolutely safe one. Whenever you try a new vaccine, you're not only taking it to protect yourself, but also to prevent the infectious agent in the community. One can argue the community has a stake in your being vaccinated. It would be tragic if as a nation we overreact and stop using vaccines or withdraw from vaccine production because of some rare adverse effects while overlooking the benefits to the majority. When people in Great Britain did just that recently there was a recurrence of disease previously controlled by vaccines, including new cases of paralytic polio.[24]

There is also the problem of testing the vaccine on humans. It is unlikely that healthy volunteers will be breaking down the doors of research labs to try out a vaccine that could conceivably infect them, and there is no point in testing a protective agent in someone who is already infected. Researchers are hopeful, however, that some people will want to serve as human guinea pigs, and the scientists running the U.S. vaccine trial have recruited sixty healthy homosexual volunteers who have no trace of the virus or AIDS antibodies in their blood and whose sexual behavior places them at low risk.

Members of high-risk groups not yet infected might also be wary of serving as guinea pigs, for even though they ostensibly would be buying insurance, those who have adopted safer lifestyles may see no advantage in taking a chance when they might be preventing the disease themselves through their altered behavior.

Moreover, both the high-risk volunteers and the researchers who administer the test vaccine would face a dilemma that is not an issue when the experimentation is performed in animals. In animal tests, a chimp, say, would get the vaccine, then a shot of AIDS virus to see if protection results. To really test a vaccine in a member of a high-risk group, the person would have to get the serum, then would have to be expected to continue doing the very things that are known to cause AIDS: shooting up drugs with shared needles and engaging in anal sex with an infected partner. Counseling such behavior, even expecting it, is really akin to deliberately injecting the AIDS virus into a human volunteer. No researcher today could or would inoculate someone with virulent material to see if that person was immune, as Edward Jenner did:

> John Phillips, a Tradesman of this town, had the Cow Pox at so early a period as nine years of age. At the age of sixty-two I inoculated him, and was very careful in selecting matter in its most active state. It was taken from the arm of a boy just before the commencement of the eruptive fever, and instantly inserted. It very speedily produced a stinglike feel in the part. An efflorescence appeared, which on the fourth day was rather extensive, and some degree of pain and stiffness were felt about the shoulder; but on the fifth day these symptoms began to disappear, and in a day or two after went entirely off, without producing any effect on the system.[25]

Finally, there is the time it must take to determine whether a vaccine is truly effective: if the latency period of AIDS is as long as it is believed to be, there will be many years of waiting before anyone can be sure a vaccine really works.

Simply developing a vaccine, therefore, does not end the AIDS story. For beyond determining just how to test it safely and prove its effectiveness — formidable obstacles in their own right — are other difficult questions that would arise once a vaccine is available: Who gets it and at what age? Should vaccination be entirely voluntary, or mandatory for high-risk groups only, or required for the general population? Should vaccination be a condition for employment, marriage, or travel? Should minors be allowed to have the vaccine on demand without parental approval? Should a person who has been vaccinated have to reveal that fact?

There are no easy answers, and indeed one might make a case for forgetting about a vaccine, given the difficulties in preparing, testing, and administering one. It may be argued that venereal diseases usually peak out at a certain percentage of the population, and that perhaps the AIDS virus — far less efficient than certain other organisms, which, despite their lethality, have not been able to wipe out humankind — simply has to run its course, while we try to develop drugs to treat it, and rely on public education, safe sex, and carefully screened blood supplies to prevent it. But then again, who can say? As epidemiologist June Osborn of the University of Michigan put it:

> We must keep in mind that the AIDS virus is a new pathogen; although the general trend of new human microbes is thought to be toward settling down and domesticating further, we have almost no experience to justify that theoretical expectation. On evolutionary grounds, it behooves a successful parasite not to "make waves," and with that in mind one could argue that the new virus is likely to become less transmissible and less virulent. But evolution takes a very long time, and humanity has known this virus for less than 30 years.[26]

12

Preventing AIDS

The risk of becoming infected with the AIDS virus does not have to do with being a homosexual man or being a member of any group. The risk for AIDS is a behavior, having sex with someone who is infected, or being exposed to blood that is infected.

— *Dr. Anthony Fauci*

GIVEN THE OBSTACLES IN THE WAY of developing a vaccine that will prevent AIDS, current efforts to limit its spread are wholly dependent upon making behavioral changes if one is in a high-risk group, and, if one is not, on taking precautions to avoid contact with the virus. Because the virus is not transmitted casually, and because it enters the body in very specific ways, whether or not AIDS is acquired becomes virtually a personal decision.

Health professionals, gay organizations, and drug treatment centers have established the following guidelines in an effort to control the disease.

Practice Safe Sex
Since the vast majority of AIDS cases and infections have occurred among sexually active homosexual men, and are expected to continue to do so, much of the advice on how to avoid infection has been aimed in their direction, although some of the suggestions obviously apply to heterosexuals as well.

• Avoid multiple or anonymous sexual partners (or both), having sex with anyone who has had such partners, partners who are or might be infected with the AIDS virus, and partners of those who have had sex with an AIDS-infected individual. Asking about a prospective partner's sexual history may be one way of thwarting trouble, but as someone has said, the question begs for a lie.

• Avoid receptive and insertive anal intercourse, dangerous practices such as fisting and rimming (anal kissing), and contact with a partner's semen, blood, feces, or urine.

• Do not share dildos or other insertive objects. They can transfer the virus to the site, or they may force virus already in the rectal area into the bloodstream through abrasions caused by friction.

• Do not have sexual contact with individuals who use IV drugs; this includes open-mouthed kissing, because even though the risk is low, the AIDS virus has been found in saliva; if mouth lesions or infections are present, especially sores or bleeding gums, the risk of exposure to AIDS is increased. (This advice applies to homosexual women as well. Although lesbians are far less apt to contract any venereal disease, and though there have been but two reported cases of female-to-female transmission of AIDS, some health professionals think that such transmission between an infected and a noninfected woman is theoretically possible through deep kissing, amorous biting, oral-genital sex, or through use of a shared dildo.)

• Avoid oral sex with an infected or high-risk partner and, if infected, do not engage in the practice with someone else. Infected semen is rich in virus, and while some studies have shown that the AIDS virus does not appear to be readily transmitted through oral sex, the practice may be dangerous, especially if infected, ejaculated semen gets into mouth sores. A person fighting a gum infection or flu is more at risk, apparently, because in such circumstances the lungs normally shed virus-favored T-4 cells into the mouth to help fight off the infection. (If infected semen is swallowed, according to researchers, there is probably little risk, since the virus presumably would be inactivated in the stomach by bacterial enzymes.) Oral sex can also spread syphilis, gonorrhea, and herpes, and these venereal infections can predispose someone to AIDS.

• Use condoms and spermicide. Studies have demonstrated that antibodies to the AIDS virus were much more likely to develop in people who did not use barrier methods, or used them infrequently. Although condoms frequently fail — some experts say the failure rate is 10 percent per user over a year, and perhaps as much as 20 percent — they undoubtedly will help curb the spread of AIDS. Virologist Jay Levy of the University of California at San Francisco recently tested the effectiveness of condoms by filling them with a fluid containing a high concentration of AIDS virus, then waiting to see if the virus passed through. Even after three weeks, there was no evidence that it had done so. Condoms should, however, be latex, since these are safer than those made from "natural" material, such as lambskin. One problem with condoms, though, is that they can break, and chances are that if they do, it will be during anal sex, a far more traumatic act than vaginal intercourse.

"There is no evidence that the standard condom membrane will stand up to anal sex," said a 1986 report in the *British Medical Journal.* "Manufacturers have concentrated on producing even finer products offering high sensitivity and only now are beginning to produce condoms especially for prophylactic use. A French firm with a British agent, for example, has produced what it claims is a tougher condom, and a firm in the north of England will market early next year a self-sealing condom to safeguard against spillage."[1]

Insofar as spermicide is concerned, nonoxynol-9, as mentioned earlier, has proved that it can kill the AIDS virus in test tubes. (It is also used in some lubricants, so-called female hygiene products, and diaper wipes.) It works by bursting the outer coat of sperm and of several disease organisms, and it appears to be safe on the skin and vagina, as well as when ingested in small amounts during oral sex. But, again, there is no proof that spermicide, or condoms, will always prevent transmission of the AIDS virus during sex. "Some say," noted Clark Taylor, a professor at the Institute for the Advanced Study of Human Sexuality in San Francisco, "that the only safe sex is no sex at all, or a monogamous relationship with someone who has been abstinent since 1978."[2]

• Avoid the use of inhaled volatile nitrites ("poppers"), such as amyl and isobutyl, as well as opiates like heroin. Although, as we have seen, their role in the development of AIDS is unclear, there is at least a suspicion that they may contribute to immunosuppression.

• Do not douche before or after sex. Doing so can weaken the natural defense against infection.

• Do not use petroleum jelly or similar products as rectal or vaginal lubricants; they can trap germs and irritate the mucous membranes. Use water-based gels instead.

• Find alternatives. "To prevent AIDS," advises the Safer Sex Committee of New York, a coalition of concerned gays, physicians, psychologists, and other health professionals that takes an extremely explicit stance on the matter,

> we must change the ways we have sex. Our great gay imaginations can help us make these changes. Some men have responded by not having sex. Others who still want to have sex with other men are realizing that great sex can be healthy sex . . . Here are some fun things you can do that are healthy: Showering together can be a real turn-on. Washing thoroughly is important before and after sex. Talking sweet, kinky, funny, dirty, butch and loving. Be creative! Touching, hugging, cuddling, stroking, caressing, massaging, even wrestling. Skin anything you like that doesn't break the skin. For a lot of men, nipples are just as erotic as asses and cocks. Erotica uniforms, drag, leather, hot porn, jock straps, posing and safe S/M scenes. Jacking off yourself, each other and in jack-off clubs. Rubbing lubricant anywhere on his body or yours. Try fucking between your partner's thighs.

Has there been any noticeable alteration in sexual behavior among gays, and if so, has the change had any effect on halting the spread of AIDS?

Many gays are aware that the pool of infected individuals is already a frighteningly large one, and that therefore their risk of contracting the disease from someone is still high, even though they may themselves change their behavior. Many are concerned that their past behavior may already have placed them at considerable risk. Most are also quite aware that the steps leading from initial infection to AIDS are still obscure. Some are still undoubtedly hoping against hope that science will discover a cure or a preventive vaccine. Thus, not all gay men feel they have any control over their future health status, and some men have considerable doubt as to the value of changing their current sexual practices.

Still, there are indications that a growing number of others are practicing safer sex, and a number of studies are confirming that the cautionary words are being heeded. At the University of Michigan, Jill Joseph of the School of Public Health examined the behavior patterns of 978 homosexual men in Chicago who had a mean age of 34.6 years and an average of 16.5 years of homosexual experience. They answered a self-administered questionnaire about their knowledge of AIDS, their perceptions of vulnerability, and whether they thought changing their behavior would reduce the risk of contracting the disease. Eighty percent of 909 respondents said they had modified their behavior in some way since the AIDS epidemic began, mainly by reducing the number of sexual partners they had.

When asked about behavior changes during the month preceding the questionnaire, just over half reported having no contact with an anonymous partner. Half also reported having no receptive anal sex; of those who did, one in five were modifying their behavior by using condoms.[3] (Gay males, traditionally, have avoided the use of condoms, since they have come to represent straight sexual practices, and because one of the principal reasons for using them, contraception, does not apply.)

Another study, conducted in Atlanta by Roger Bakeman of Georgia State University, also corroborated the widespread anecdotal evidence that gay men's behavior has been changing dramatically in response to AIDS. When Bakeman asked a racially and educationally diverse group of gay males whether, and how, their sexual behavior had changed, 57 percent said they had reduced their number of partners, and 59 percent said they had changed their sexual practices. Interestingly, safer sex practices were more prevalent among those who did not have lovers, who had attended safe-sex seminars, and who were more educated. "These men have heard the message," Bakeman reported to the American Psychological Association's annual convention in 1986. "More importantly, the majority have changed their behavior as well. Why men with lovers are more likely to engage in unsafe practices is unclear. Perhaps certain practices are expected between lovers, perhaps lovers think they are less at risk. Whatever the reason, these results suggest that some educational efforts should target lovers specifically."[4]

Have the behavioral changes had any impact on AIDS? Again, no one can say for sure, although experts point to a study showing a decline in the number of new infections among previously uninfected individuals — notably in San Francisco — as proof that changes in behavior have helped. "We believe that the best explanation for the declining seroconversion rates is the substantial reduction in the numbers of receptive anal/genital contacts with ejaculation," concluded epidemiologist Warren Winkelstein of the University of California at Berkeley, who led the study.

But as optimistic as the findings were, there was a somber side. At least 18,000 homosexual/bisexual men live in the study area, and approximately 9,000 have now been infected with the AIDS virus; many of them — at least 15 percent — may develop AIDS over the next five years. Thus, while there have been dramatic changes in sexual practices in the San Francisco area, the actual number of AIDS cases is still increasing, and certain segments of the gay community are so saturated with the virus that it no longer takes hundreds of sexual contacts to risk infection.

"It's a very major risk to enter these communities," warned June Osborn. "So the fifteen- or sixteen-year-old kid who's going to declare his same-sex preference should understand that there's a serious chance of infection that can truly be a matter of life and death. The false hope of a vaccine or a cure prevents people from examining their sexual options. False hopes keep people from having to face up to the fact that prevention is the most rational thing, and it is possible — not easy, but possible."[5]

Terminate a Drug Habit

Changing established sexual habits or learning to practice monogamy and celibacy are difficult to accomplish. But for many people, alternative ways of obtaining sexual gratification are available and changes can be made.

Not so for the intravenous-drug addict, who generally must adopt the addict's version of celibacy — kicking the habit altogether — if he or she wants to be sure of avoiding AIDS. Thus, the main piece of advice given to IV-drug abusers is to get professional help in terminating the habit. If they cannot kick it, they are advised to avoid sharing needles and syringes (boiling them does not ensure sterility), something that is not always that easy to do, given the fact that many street dealers often reseal previously used needles and sell them for new. Also, sharing needles is universal. It is associated with initiation into the drug cult, may be a social-bonding mechanism, and is done for practical reasons: drug users often do not have enough money to buy an unused needle, may be fearful of being arrested if they carry their own paraphernalia, or merely cannot find unused equipment.

Thus, from the standpoint of behavioral psychology, IV-drug abuse, with its gnawing compulsion and unstable life-style, is probably the most difficult behavior pattern to change permanently. It is probably for that reason that the controversial alternative known as "needle exchange" has been suggested by some medical experts. It would involve distributing free, sterile syringes to addicts in return for the dirty needles they are now using, a practice under way in Amsterdam since 1984 (where only two AIDS cases have been diagnosed among addicts thus far) and Australia. Support for a test program came recently from the CDC's James Curran, who remarked, "I would not discount anything in trying to combat this disease. The problem we face is bigger than politics."[6]

Needle exchange seems a valid approach, considering that IV-drug abusers are the second-largest group to have developed AIDS in the United States, that they play a role in the heterosexual transmission of the disease, and that drug-abusing women can pass the disease along to their fetuses. The enormity of the problem is underlined by the situation in New Jersey, where nearly 60 percent of the AIDS cases are drug-related, a higher percentage than in any other state. Studies suggest that more than half the addicts in northern New Jersey have been exposed to the virus; thus anyone sharing a needle even once has a better than 50-percent chance of being exposed as well.[7] Needless to say, the proposal has run into strong opposition. The reason is fairly obvious: the state would be encouraging drug use and creating more addicts, a greater threat to the public health than AIDS.

Given the general reluctance of state legislatures to go along with the proposal, behavior modification, as difficult as it is among addicts, seems to be the only viable approach. Indeed, it may eventually work with more education. "There is a stereo-typical notion that IV drug users are so driven by their habits that they have no regard for the health consequences of injecting drugs," observed the National Academy of Sciences' Institute of Medicine in its 1986 report on AIDS.

> This stereotype is accompanied by a view of IV drug users as a homogeneous group, although in fact people from all walks of life use IV drugs, some on an occasional basis. Research on IV drug users in New York City, however, clearly shows that concern about dying from AIDS is great enough to change the behavior of many drug users. One study of patients in methadone treatment found that more than 90 percent knew that AIDS was transmitted through sharing injection equipment. Of these patients, 59 percent reported behavior change to reduce their risk of contracting AIDS. Other studies have confirmed this finding, with the most common behavior changes including increased use of sterile needles, reductions in sharing equipment, and reductions in drug injection.[8]

General Precautions
Even if you do not abuse IV drugs, are not a homosexual or a bisexual male who practices anal sex, and do not have sex with anonymous or multiple partners, infected persons, or prosti-tutes, there is always the possibility, unlikely though it might

be, that you could become infected with the AIDS virus. But that risk would be present only if you were intimately exposed to infected blood or body fluids, or both, through deep accidental cuts or, if you are a health care worker or researcher, through needle-sticks.

Some occupations and practices entail higher risk than others. Included in this category are "invasive" operative procedures, the kind that require entry into tissues, cavities, and organs; surgeons who perform cesarean deliveries and nurses who assist in the procedure must, for example, take special care when handling the placenta, and even the infant, until blood and amniotic fluid have been removed from its skin; dental procedures that involve cutting or removal of oral tissues or teeth — any that draw blood — can also be risky. Apart from surgeons, nurses, and dental workers, among others at some risk are hospital aides, lab technicians, hospital cleaning and housekeeping staff, laundry workers, incinerator attendants, sterilization and supply staff, morgue attendants, ambulance personnel, police and firefighters, and sewage workers.

Here are some general guidelines that fall under the heading of simple common sense:

• Do not handle or use razors, toothbrushes, or other implements that could be contaminated with blood and that have been used by someone with AIDS or someone who might have been exposed to the virus.

• For health care workers: If you handle blood or body fluids, or must touch mucous membranes (in the mouth, for example), wear gloves; in addition, a mask and protective eyewear should be worn if you are conducting procedures (such as centrifuging, blending, or respiratory therapy care) where an aerosol is created; if widespread soiling is expected, wear a gown. If you are dealing with patients, gloves should be changed between all patient contacts. If a glove is torn or a needle-stick or other injury occurs, the glove must be changed as soon as possible, and the needle or instrument removed.

No health care worker who has oozing lesions, or so-called weeping dermatitis, should perform or assist in any invasive procedure, or handle any equipment used for patient care. Finally, frequent hand washing is an obvious, but very effective, means of preventing the spread of the virus. (More-detailed guidelines for health care workers are contained in the April 11, 1986, *Morbidity and Mortality Weekly Report* of the Centers for Disease Control; and for health care workers and others in the risk occupations listed above, from the Service Employees International Union, AFL-CIO, Washington, D.C.)

• If you have a positive AIDS blood test, do not donate blood, sperm, or organs, and consider postponing pregnancy.

13

When Someone Has AIDS

THE BEST PROTECTION AGAINST AIDS is, as outlined in the previous chapter, careful behavior. But there is a danger that that advice will be translated into avoidance behavior: avoidance of those who have AIDS. While the spread of the disease can be stopped by avoiding intimate contact with the virus, the disease will not be stopped by shunning the person with AIDS. Such callous neglect can break down any psychological defense mechanisms the patient may have constructed, and can only enhance his or her already intense fear and anxiety.

Just as there are guidelines about how to prevent spread of AIDS, so, too, are there guidelines about how to prevent the spread of helplessness and emotional shock in those already infected. Although the following suggestions were meant primarily for the gay community, they are relevant to all who are seriously ill with AIDS or with any other life-threatening illness. They have been summarized and adapted from a brochure prepared by the Chelsea Psychotherapy Associates of Manhattan.[1] When someone has AIDS:

- Do not avoid him. Your involvement instills hope. Be the friend and the loved one you have always been. But call before you visit since he may not feel up to a visitor at that moment. Call back.
- Touch him. A simple squeeze of the hand, or a hug, can let him know you still care.

- Cry with him, laugh with him. These intimate experiences can enrich you both.
- Do not be reluctant to ask about his illness. And do not confuse his acceptance of it with defeat. Acceptance might give him a sense of his own power. Also, do not feel that you always have to talk. It is okay to sit together silently, reading, listening to music, watching television, holding hands.
- Help him feel good about his looks if possible. Tell him he looks good, but only if it is realistic to do so. If his appearance has changed, do not ignore it. Be gentle, but do not lie.
- Include him in decision making, no matter how simple or silly the decisions may seem to you. He has lost control of so many aspects of his life.
- Tell him what you would like to do for him, and if he agrees, keep any promises you make.
- Be prepared for him to get angry with you for no apparent reason, even though you have been there and done everything you could. Do not take it personally, and be flattered that he is close enough to you to risk sharing his anger and frustration.
- Do not lecture or be angry if he seems to be handling his illness in a way that you think is inappropriate. He may not be where you expect or need him to be.
- Take him for a walk after knowing his limitations; get him to his doctor; bring a favorite dish; call and ask for a shopping list; offer to help answer correspondence. Offer to do household chores, but do not do for him what he can do for himself. Ask before doing anything.
- If you are religious, ask if you could pray for or with him.
- Send a card that says simply, "I care."
- Talk about the future, tomorrow, next week, next year. Hope is vital to him.

14

AIDS Testing

WHAT IS THE AIDS TEST?

First of all, the so-called AIDS test is not a test for AIDS. Second, as is true of all diagnostic tests, it is not perfect. Approved by the Food and Drug Administration on March 2, 1985, less than a year after the AIDS virus was confirmed as the infective agent, the test was devised to determine if donated blood for transfusions has been exposed to the virus. It does this by detecting the earliest signs of seroconversion; that is, it tests for the antibodies that are produced when exposure to the AIDS virus occurs.

Formally known as an enzyme-linked immunosorbent assay (ELISA), the laboratory testing procedure begins by attaching proteins from inactivated virus to a plastic sheet or plastic beads. Serum from a blood donor is added, and if the donor is infected with AIDS virus, the antibodies made against it will bind to the protein antigens stuck to the plastic. The last steps involve confirming the presence of antibodies by a process that produces a color reaction when they are encountered, then measuring the degree of positivity.

The term that is used when antibodies are discovered, *seropositive*, means that the individual whose blood has been tested has at some time been infected by the AIDS virus. Actual identification of the AIDS virus, the most definitive indication that a person has been infected, is a laborious lab procedure that

requires isolating the virus from peripheral leukocytes, monocytes, and macrophages in the blood; from bone marrow, lymph
nodes, and the thymus gland; from macrophages in the brain;
from the epithelial and endothelial cells in the cornea of the
eye; and from cells or cell-free fluids from semen, cervical fluids,
saliva, tears, cerebrospinal fluid, urine, and plasma.

DOES A POSITIVE ANTIBODY TEST
MEAN YOU HAVE AIDS?

First, we have to define what is meant by "positive." According
to the Public Health Service, the term describes a repeatably
reactive sample that has been determined to contain antibody
by a more specific, supplementary test. Only then may a person
be termed seropositive.

Once that positive finding is established, the following may
be said:

- The person is infected with HIV.
- Most persons infected will be infected for life.
- All persons who are antibody-positive, whether they
  are symptom-free or ill, must be considered to be potentially infectious to others by sexual transmission, by
  sharing of drug injection equipment, by childbearing,
  or by donation of blood, semen, or organs.
- Antibody-positivity is not synonomous with having AIDS.
  However, by the best current estimates, 35 percent of
  HIV-antibody-positive persons may experience progression to AIDS over six to eight years.
- No one can predict precisely who among antibody-
  positive persons will be ill or fatally ill in the future,
  nor is it possible to prevent such outcomes.
- All antibody-positive persons should seek information
  and advice on how to protect their sexual contacts and
  future children from infection.

On the other hand, although the results of an ELISA test are
reasonably accurate even without confirmatory testing, a single

test cannot automatically establish that a person is infected. It is possible that a positive test may result from exposure to viruses other than the AIDS virus; for instance, researchers have discovered that patients suffering from both alcoholism and liver-damaging hepatitis-B virus often test positive for the AIDS virus but show no evidence of such infection when retested with more definitive laboratory procedures.

Thus, simply testing with ELISA is not enough, for despite its high degree of sensitivity — and ELISA was deliberately made so, in order to catch virtually every scrap of blood that genuinely contains antibodies — its predictive value ranges from very good, in cases involving individuals at increased risk of AIDS-virus infection, to very poor in those of unknown or low risk of infection.

This raises the issue of false positives: those test results that wrongly indicate the presence of AIDS-virus antibodies in patients' and donors' blood or semen, perhaps because of bacterial contamination, poor quality of a test sample, or technical problems that can arise during the testing procedure. Most ELISA false-positive readings are just over the line of the test for positivity, while most "true" positives — those that can be confirmed by actually isolating the AIDS virus — are usually several times higher than the positive threshold.

It is estimated that out of any given sample of blood donors who test positive on a single ELISA, half to two-thirds may be false positives. This is so because uninfected persons — who are vastly more numerous than infected ones — sometimes give off positive reactions due to the sensitivity of the test. (Sensitivity varies considerably from manufacturer to manufacturer among the dozen or so licensed test kits, and even among different lots from the same manufacturer.) This small fraction of the uninfected donors produces many more of the positive reactions than arise from the few people actually infected with the virus. That is, the odds are great that any single ELISA-positive reading comes from an uninfected person. Low positive values are often not reproducible, however, and repeated, independent samples from an uninfected donor whose first test was positive will likely turn up negative.

Generally, ELISA-positive blood is retested with a more sensitive, although time-consuming, antibody test called Western Blot — a method that is considered the current "gold standard" for AIDS-virus testing and that can sometimes suggest whether the infection is a recent or an old one.

But as reassuring as some of that may sound, any positive readings should not be taken lightly. For one thing, the sensitivity of the ELISA kits for the AIDS virus is such that it does turn up the antibodies when they are present, and since AIDS kills, a positive reading, even with the chance it is false, rightfully raises a red flag. Moreover, it has to be mentioned that the follow-up tests are not perfect, either. If an ELISA-positive individual retests as negative and sees his rather heartening "second opinion" as a license to give blood, he or she may still be putting recipients at risk, albeit a small one.

In the past year or two, screening agencies have been discarding all blood that is antibody-positive after repeat testing. To further minimize the risk, when a blood sample comes up ELISA-positive and Western Blot–negative, blood banks throw the blood away as a precautionary measure and place the donor's name in a "donor deferral" registry, which means the individual's blood will not be used in the future. This is done even though a donor who tests both positive and negative is considered uninfected, and is usually not notified. (An NIH panel has recommended, however, that such individuals be informed of their test results, and told, furthermore, that it is unlikely they carry the AIDS virus.)

The person with proven antibodies, of course, makes the call for caution even louder. For one thing, researchers believe that with a retrovirus like the AIDS virus, chances are that once a person is truly infected he will carry the virus with him for the rest of his life; it does not just hit the cells and then slip quietly out of the body. Also, no one knows exactly how many individuals who unequivocally test positive for AIDS antibodies will go on to develop the disease. Some experts, such as those at Baylor College of Medicine, use the example of the TB bacterium, which is present in about 10 million people, or 4 percent of the U.S. population. Except for about 5 percent of those who have the bacterium, these people do not have tuberculosis, they are not going to get the disease, nor are they going to give it to anyone else.[1]

But the realistic current estimates are that 35 percent of those with positive readings will contract AIDS, while another 25 percent will develop ARC. Given the unusual and deadly nature of AIDS, and given the current gaps in what is known about the disease and the limitations inherent in the current testing methods, the assumption must be that anyone with proven antibodies, whether or not the individual has symptoms of AIDS, is capable of passing on the disease to others through its well-defined pathways into the body. And another point bears repeating: anyone with proven antibodies has to be regarded as infectious — and since the virus is a tenacious one, that means infectious for life, even though some carriers remain healthy.

Without doubt, antibodies to the virus usually turn up in the blood of those with AIDS or AIDS-related conditions. In one study, 82 percent of 88 patients with AIDS tested positive, 16 percent were borderline, and only 2 percent were negative. By contrast, only 1 percent of volunteer blood donors were positive, 6 percent were borderline, and 93 percent were negative.[2] The antibodies are also present in many people who are members of the high-risk groups. (In New York City, 60 percent to 80 percent of intravenous-drug users, many of them homosexuals, reportedly have antibodies to the AIDS virus.)

That the presence of antibodies in an individual means the AIDS virus has not disappeared from his body is a view shared by most researchers. Some estimate that more than two-thirds of seropositive individuals (if not all) carry live, infectious virus, probably because the antibody is incapable of fully neutralizing it and, thus, does not rid the body of infection. Robert Gallo's group at the NCI has claimed that it can isolate the virus from the blood of more than 80 percent of individuals with observable antibodies.

Scientists are refining the AIDS tests to make them more accurate, and already have come up with some very promising results. Current approaches include developing tests that would screen for the virus's protein by-products, rather than the antibodies produced against it, or that would detect the virus itself. These methods would, of course, provide a more definite diagnosis of infection because they would spot those individuals who currently slip through the screening system because they do not immediately mount an immune reaction (ELISA, for instance, cannot detect patients in the very early infection period), and would confirm whether the virus is present in an individual who does produce antibodies.

Two U.S. firms, Dupont and Abbott Diagnostics, have each developed kits that detect the virus itself by locating a protein, p24, nestled in the viral core. Apparently, however, the kits are cumbersome, and require several hours to yield results. "There is a heightened need for an ultra-sensitive and cost-effective means of quickly measuring the [AIDS] virus and its antigens directly," observed Dr. Fred Fraser of Dupont's biomedical-products department.

> From what researchers have learned so far about variations in the course and appearance of antibodies in the AIDS disease and its sub-clinical conditions, we should expect that during asymptomatic states, there may be a period ranging from several weeks to months when a state of viremia [virus in the blood] exists with no significant antibody present, and it will take a test system for direct measurement of the virus and viral by-products that has sensitivity considerably beyond what's achievable today to efficiently test for the presence of virus.[3]

It would also enable researchers to better evaluate drugs aimed at eliminating the virus from a patient.

Coming up with an easy, direct test for finding virus in the blood is, however, difficult, because the AIDS virus is so often present at extremely low levels: it perhaps hides for years in just 1 of every 500,000 white blood cells. There have been some rather promising developments. Researchers at the University of California at San Francisco have, for example, come up with a colorimetric method (known as "competition ELISA") for detecting very low levels of the AIDS virus in infected cells and body fluids, notably blood. The procedure measures specifically the amount of the major structural protein of the virus by its ability to compete against a highly purified form of the same protein that has been produced by recombinant-DNA technology. The technique can apparently detect as few as 100 infected cells, or 10 picograms (10 billionths of a milligram) of viral protein per test sample, with very low risk of false-positive results.

In another effort to spot the elusive virus, several companies have developed promising methods that make use of what is known as DNA probe technology. Although the scientific description of how one example of it works is formidable ("The method involves amplification of viral nucleic acid sequences by a technique called polymerase chain reaction and rapid detection of the sequences by a technique called oligomer restriction analysis," says one technical account in *Chemical and Engineering News*),[4] what it all amounts to is fairly straightforward: instead of detecting antibodies to the virus, as the current tests do, the chemically synthesized probe, actually constructed of selected bits of DNA, latches on to the DNA that the AIDS virus has copied from its RNA when the virus infects a cell; radioactive or chemical tags on the probe "illuminate" the viral DNA, which is then read by imaging techniques.

In one of the probe systems under development (by Cetus Corporation of Emeryville, California), the target DNA, even if present in tiny amounts in a suspected sample of blood, is cloned to produce something on the order of a million copies; the duplicating process makes it far easier to identify the DNA segment that betrays the virus. Thus far, the Cetus studies have turned up AIDS virus in infected cells, and at this writing tests are under way on blood and semen samples taken from AIDS victims.

Another probe, under development at Enzo Biochem, Inc., in New York City, uses a radioactive tag stronger than conventional ones; this, in effect, boosts the probe's detecting power, enabling it to find the virus more easily in infected cells and blood samples. According to Dr. Elazar Rabbani, Enzo's chairman and president,

> The inaccurate results of the [current] antibody tests may lead to improper patient treatment, unnecessary disposal of huge quantities of uncontaminated blood supplies, and

the use of AIDS-contaminated blood in transfusions. We believe that our test could correct all these inaccuracies. The tests, which enable early AIDS detection, will initially assist in preventing the spread of AIDS through early diagnosis, and will lead to better management of the patient and the disease. The DNA-based tests also eliminate potential hazardous exposure of medical technicians to the live virus. Unlike present antibody and culture-based tests that require handling of the live virus by technicians, ours are performed on clinical samples which have been treated to kill the virus.[5]

HOW SAFE IS THE NATION'S BLOOD SUPPLY?

In general, one might say that the supply is very safe. According to CDC epidemiologists, the chance now of a blood recipient's getting the virus is less than 1 in 100,000 (of the 12 million or so units of whole blood donated every year in the United States, that amounts to around 120 virus-contaminated units), far lower than the risk of death from the complications of general anesthesia, which has been put at around 1 in 10,000. Fewer than 2 percent of AIDS cases are thought to be transmitted by blood transfusion. Such favorable odds, CDC officials believe, should not deter the 1 out of every 100 persons in the United States who will have to receive blood this year during surgery or some other medical procedure.

However, to be honest, one should also say that the nation's blood banks are not entirely safe. Nor have they ever been so. Hepatitis B was a classic, serious complication of blood transfusions, and even though an almost foolproof screening test for HBV has been widely used for more than fifteen years, new forms of hepatitis caused by yet-unidentified viruses have surfaced, and are believed to be infecting 7 percent to 10 percent of the 4 million Americans who receive transfusions every year. If true, this would be a far greater threat than transfusion-related AIDS. Transfusion can also pass along one of the five members of the human herpes group, the cytomegalovirus (CMV), a slow-spreading agent that can cause a mononucleosislike illness, birth defects, and infections in patients whose immune systems have been suppressed.

Those who have contracted AIDS through blood transfusions (among them are 15 percent of the infants and children diagnosed with the disease) may have contracted it before the nation's blood-collection agencies began their screening programs. But even with a far safer blood supply, there remains the possibility of false negatives: the failure to detect antibody to the AIDS virus, perhaps because the test was done too early in a suspected carrier (there is a "window" of two weeks to six months between the time of exposure to the virus and the development of antibodies), or because of some failure in the test itself or in the processing of samples. Although far less common than false positives, false negatives are, still, a matter for some concern. Part of the problem lies with the dominant antigen — the p24, or gag, antigen — that is bound to the test's beads. For some unexplained reason, antibody titers to the antigen decline in many patients as they develop AIDS, and because of this, ELISA misses a substantial number of patients with AIDS.

A 1986 report on a study by Dr. Alfred J. Saah of the National Institute of Allergy and Infectious Diseases, and his colleagues at several institutions, attests to the discrepancies in the reactivity of some blood specimens when tested with various ELISA kits. Dr. Saah's group had been analyzing the results of tests conducted on the blood of participants in a prospective study of 4,955 initially healthy homosexual and bisexual men in four cities. The ongoing study, known as the Multicenter AIDS Cohort Study (MACS), is designed to trace the natural history of infection with the AIDS virus in these men. Participants are seen every six months, blood is collected at each visit, and testing is done with various commercially available ELISA kits and Western Blot tests.

Dr. Saah's analysis of the data revealed that some blood specimens identified as antibody-negative by certain kits were antibody-positive when tested with kits from different manufacturers and with Western Blots. The Western Blots showed that these specimens contained antibodies to core proteins of the AIDS virus, and frequently lacked antibodies to envelope proteins. (Antibodies to core proteins are often the first antibodies to show up during early infection with the virus. It should be pointed out that tests of subsequent specimens showed increased production of antibodies to both core and envelope proteins, reflecting a true infection with the AIDS virus. The ELISA kits of all manufacturers identified these later specimens with greater accuracy.)

Dr. Saah acknowledged that all homosexual and bisexual males have been advised to refrain from donating blood, but said it was not possible to measure the effects of the advisory. "It is now apparent," he said, "that a certain proportion of potential blood donors with very early infection lack sufficient levels of antibody to envelope proteins and thus will be missed by all of the currently licensed test kits." (In the study, of 30 specimens that were positive for core antibody only, kits from one company identified 2, one from another, 4, and still another, 13. The kits of two companies identified 25 each, indicating that the sensitivity of at least some of the ELISA kits to core-protein antibodies still has to be enhanced.)

Compounding the danger of false negatives is the fact that a few infected individuals do not make antibodies for a prolonged period even though they actively carry the infection — a phenomenon believed to occur in less than 1 percent. There is also a slim possibility that if the AIDS epidemic spreads beyond the known risk groups, the blood of the new, infected groups may not have the same markers that are now geared to the current tests. It has been estimated that 5 percent of all antibody-test results presently fail to turn up evidence of the virus in patients where the virus is, indeed, known to be present through other means.

One study, published in 1984 in the British medical journal *The Lancet*, found that 4 out of 96 individuals in whom the AIDS virus had been detected were without any symptoms of the disease and, moreover, had no detectable antibodies — a peculiarity that would have enabled them to slip through the current AIDS test. Another study, at the Pennsylvania State University School of Medicine, looked at a group of apparently healthy wives of hemophiliacs and discovered, through a tedious laboratory procedure, that 6 were carrying the AIDS virus, probably contracted through having sex with their infected husbands. However, an AIDS screening test produced no sign of antibodies to the virus for some eleven months after detection of the virus in their blood.

Perhaps the most dramatic example of the ELISA test's failure involved a thirty-one-year-old blood donor in Colorado who had given blood so soon after a homosexual contact that he had yet to develop antibodies. The donor tested negative for the AIDS virus in April of 1985, and donated again in August, about three months after he began having sex, without using condoms, with a homosexual, the donor's first such contact in eleven years. That blood, too, tested negative. But a sixty-year-old, apparently heterosexual surgical patient picked up the virus after being transfused with the blood donated in August. In November, the donor once again gave blood, but this time it showed signs of antibodies and was discarded. Another patient, according to the CDC, received the same blood donated in August, and he, too, contracted an AIDS-virus infection, although in that instance health authorities could not say for sure whether the transfusion was to blame since the recipient was a homosexual who reported that he had had sex with several partners.

As Harvard's Max Essex, who contributed greatly to developing the ELISA antibody test, has put it, "I'm not saying the test we have now should not be used, or that it hasn't greatly cut the odds of contracting AIDS through transfusion. But I'm afraid these overly optimistic statements that are being made about the safety of the blood supply will eliminate public pressure to develop better tests."[6]

Besides the possibility of a batch of false-negative blood slipping through the current screening process and causing infection with the AIDS virus, there is the probability that a relatively large number of people — estimates range between 2,500 and 5,000 — got transfused blood taken from donors before the antibody test was in use, donors who later tested positive. (In July of 1986, the Greater New York Blood Program announced that it was trying to identify some 700 individuals who, since 1977, had received blood that may have been contaminated with the AIDS virus. More than 2.7 million people have received transfusions from the center since the year that AIDS is suspected to have first begun its spread in the area.) The thought is not a pleasant one, especially for the recipients, who have been receiving warning letters from their doctors under the "look-back" program established by the three major blood-collection agencies — the American Red Cross, which collects half of all blood donated in the United States (6 million units); the American Association of Blood Banks (3 million units); and the Council of Community Blood Centers (2.6 million).

The recipients notified include those who received contaminated blood from donors with full-blown AIDS, as well as recipients of blood taken from donors who tested positive for AIDS antibodies but who do not have active disease. And though it is true that the risk of getting AIDS after infection is not now enormous (only after sufficient time has elapsed will it be possible to tell if all those infected will eventually develop the disease), such is not the case with the risk of acquiring an infection from AIDS-contaminated blood: indications are that there is an exceedingly high risk of infection in recipients of seropositive blood, perhaps exceeding 90 percent.

Even though only 2 percent or so of reported AIDS cases have been linked to blood transfusion and the use of an injectable plasma blood product by hemophiliacs to stop uncontrolled bleeding (some 20,000 people have the inherited blood disease in the United States), health officials are still not resting easy. For one thing, a small number of stored blood samples taken from U.S. drug addicts in 1971 and 1972 have tested positive for AIDS antibodies, an indication that the AIDS virus may have been in this country longer than suspected. For another, because it is now believed that five years is the average time between transfusion with AIDS-tainted blood and diagnosis of the disease (instead of two, as was believed earlier), many of the AIDS infections caused by transfusions given after the middle of 1981, and perhaps even earlier, have yet to surface.

Estimates are that between 80 percent and 90 percent of severe hemophiliacs who regularly receive blood products are infected with the AIDS virus (though less than 1 percent are known to be active AIDS patients), and so are many adults who received transfusions for other ills, and many children, whose estimated rate for transfusion-associated AIDS is nearly five times that of adults. Again, no one is certain just how many of those who received tainted transfusions will eventually develop the disease. (It is also important to point out here that, contrary to what many people believe, a person cannot contract AIDS by giving blood. The needles used to draw blood from a donor are new and sterile, and are discarded after use. They are not used again on another donor.)

About all one can say, then, is that the nation's current blood supply is now *essentially* free of the AIDS virus, which is heartening news for those who will require blood, but new cases of the disease linked either to transfusions with false-negative blood that has slipped through the system, or to blood given before the screening test came into being, will continue to appear for some time. The recently discovered HIV-II also poses a problem. It is not only a new strain but a special new member of the AIDS virus family, and as such enables close to half of those it infects to get past the current tests. Ignorance on the part of donors at high risk is also a matter of some concern to blood banks. In the Colorado case, the blood donor said he felt he was not at risk for infection because he had only one sexual partner. To which the CDC has replied, "Although a steady sexual relationship with a single partner is generally safer with regard to AIDS-virus infection than relationships with multiple sexual partners, men who have had sexual contact with another man since 1977 must not donate blood." (This includes those who had only a single homosexual experience.)

In the last analysis, there is little choice for a surgical patient or a hemophiliac but to use banked blood and blood products, and to trust ELISA. As James B. Hubbard, vice-president of the American Blood Commission, has put it, "Blood bankers are trying hard to make the blood supply as safe as possible. When a person needs blood, there are usually only two alternatives. One involves a transfusion. The other is to make funeral arrangements."[7]

Blood substitutes — such as synthetic red blood cells that carry oxygen to body tissues and return carbon dioxide to the lungs for excretion, and perfluorocarbons, inert compounds of fluorine and carbon that would also, in liquid form, supplant the oxygen-carrying function of bona fide blood — are years away from development for use in humans. Autologous blood donations, units drawn from and used by the same person, are becoming more common in light of the AIDS epidemic, and are the safest method of transfusion: in 1973, according to the American Association of Blood Banks, fewer than 100 institutions offered patients an opportunity to donate their blood for their own use; in 1984, there were 656. But because autologous blood must be drawn, tested, and stored in advance (in solution, it can be kept in a refrigerator for only about seven weeks), they work best for nonanemic, healthy individuals who can plan elective surgery.

The fear of transfusion-associated AIDS has also heightened interest in another alternate approach to the standard transfusion: the directed donation. Some blood banks, like Stanford University's, accept such donations, which involve blood given by a friend, a family member, or another individual for the exclusive use of a specially designated recipient. The procedure, however, is controversial, and such donations require extra handling and paperwork, increasing the cost to patients; blood banks are also afraid that if such a practice spreads, it will fuel fears about the safety of the current blood supply, and perhaps even have a devastating effect on it by drawing away regular donors who would opt to save themselves for directed donations.

There is also an ethical problem: some blood centers use directed donations as a marketing gimmick, requiring recipients to bring in two or three times more donors than are specifically needed, in order to increase the center's blood supply. Moreover, Dr. Margot S. Kruskall, a pathologist at Harvard Medical School and medical director of Boston's Beth Israel Hospital Blood Bank, argues that because the incidence of transfusion-associated AIDS is still quite low, it is difficult to prove that recipient-selected donors are less likely to transmit AIDS than volunteer blood donors. She points out, for example, that

hepatitis B surface antigen positivity has also been seen as frequently among directed donors as volunteers. Thus, directed donors may not meet recipients' expectations regarding infectivity. This may be due, in some instances, to donors being unwilling to disclose some aspects of social history, to avoid exposure and placement in an [AIDS-virus] high-risk group. Other donors may have withheld important medical history, such as hepatitis, in order to insure that they may be able to fulfill the recipient's wish to use their blood to avoid AIDS.[8]

SHOULD THE AIDS TEST BE MANDATORY?

Mindful that testing was crucial to helping stop the spread of the disease, the Public Health Service recommended in March of 1986 that all those at risk of exposure to the AIDS virus take the blood test. "The prevalence of [AIDS-virus] antibody is high in certain risk groups in the United States," said the PHS. "Since a large proportion of seropositive, asymptomatic persons have been shown to be viremic, all seropositive individuals, whether symptomatic or not, must be presumed capable of transmitting this infection. A repeatedly reactive serologic test for [the virus] has important medical, as well as public health, implications for the individual and his/her health-care provider." The PHS cautioned, however, that "careful attention must be paid to maintaining confidentiality and to protecting records from an unauthorized disclosure. The ability of health departments to assure confidentiality — and the public confidence in that ability — are crucial to efforts to increase the number of persons requesting such testing and counseling. Without appropriate confidentiality protection, anonymous testing should be considered. Persons tested anonymously would still be offered medical evaluation and counseling."

One group of healthy individuals who are strongly advised to be tested are women in high-risk groups who are considering pregnancy or who have been partners of high-risk individuals. "Given the apparently relatively high prenatal and/or perinatal transmission rate from [AIDS-virus]-infected women to offspring," says Dr. Robert T. Schooley of the Massachusetts General Hospital's infectious-disease unit, "seropositive women should not become pregnant at the present time."[9]

Soon after the test was developed, the federal government made $9.7 million available to states to help them set up testing sites. Supplemented in some places with state funds, the testing centers, which offer free blood testing and counseling, are located in storefronts in neighborhoods with large numbers of drug addicts, in VD clinics, and in hospitals. When this book was being prepared, AIDS tests were being conducted on incoming and outgoing inmates at the nation's forty-seven federal prisons; moreover, six state prison systems and seven city or county jail systems had, according to a report by the National Institute of Justice and the American Correctional Association, been screening, or were planning to screen, all inmates, all new recruits, or all inmates belonging to at least one high-risk group; most correctional institutions were performing serologic tests for AIDS-virus antibody on a limited basis. By the end of 1985, more than 1,000 testing sites for high-risk individuals were in place throughout the United States, and had provided 93,917 pretest counseling sessions. Of some 79,000 tested, 17 percent registered positive for the virus.

Here is how one state, Massachusetts, with its network of Alternative Testing Sites, handles those who want to determine their AIDS-virus status at no cost: Individuals who are interested telephone for an appointment. Although a main site is located at the Massachusetts General Hospital (MGH), subjects are given the option to be tested at any other participating location they choose. During the initial appointment, the person receives a number from a Red Cross representative; no names are exchanged. The person is counseled about the test, and informed consent is obtained if the subject wishes to proceed. Blood is then drawn to be tested at the Red Cross, and a return appointment is arranged for seven to fourteen days after the first visit.

At the next appointment, the subject is counseled again, then asked if he or she still wishes to have the results; if the results are requested, they are given to the subject in a sealed envelope. The individual may open the envelope in the presence of the counselor, or later. Additional counseling is then offered, if requested, and other referrals are made if necessary. Since no names are exchanged and Red Cross employees rather than MGH personnel perform the test, no record of either the visit or the test result is entered in the subject's medical record. The current waiting period for Alternative Testing Site appointments is three weeks, but considerations of confidentiality and cost may make the wait worthwhile for the so-called worried well individual.

At the present time, no state allows public health officials to require antibody testing, although there have been suggestions that it be made mandatory. The Pentagon has already taken steps in this direction: in the summer of 1985, it decided to require blood screening of all new military recruits and, subsequently, added all active-duty and reserve personnel to the list. Under the rules, recruits who test positive are not allowed into the military, and active-duty personnel with positive readings are to be dismissed on medical disability if evidence of the actual disease is found; if with a positive reading there are no signs of disease, chances are the serviceman will draw a limited-duty assignment that excludes duty overseas. The military reasons that such measures are essential to protect the health of its armed forces and that of the sexual partners of its personnel here and abroad, and to ensure that battlefield blood donations will be free of the AIDS virus.

Thus far, the results of the military's testing program seem to justify the concept. Out of 3 million tested for AIDS antibodies since October of 1985, 1.6 of every 1,000 men had been exposed to the virus; for women, the rate was 0.6 per 1,000. Among those from the New York metropolitan area, the rate was 8 of 1,000 male applicants and 6 of 1,000 female; older recruits who were screened were more likely to have antibodies (presumably because they had had more sexual exposure), and there were more positive readings among recruits from the West

Coast and the East Coast from New York southward, with fewer from New England and the Mountain and upper Middle Western states.

Mandatory testing is a thorny issue. One of the chief arguments against it, of course, is that evidence of infection with the virus does not necessarily mean the fatal disease will result, or that an infected individual is irresponsible and poses a threat to society; even if someone does carry the AIDS virus, he or she cannot pass it along through casual contact, so one has to ask what purpose identifying potentially infectious individuals will serve. Another argument against it is that mandatory testing may infringe on individual rights, and that those who test positive may be discriminated against.

It appears at this stage of the AIDS epidemic that the issue of mandatory testing can only be resolved situationally, and only after carefully balancing the best interests of the community against the civil rights of individuals — the public's need for protection versus the AIDS patient's right to privacy. "The legality of measures to control the spread of infectious diseases is determined under principles of constitutional law that require the individual's interest in liberty and privacy to be balanced against the public's interest in health and safety," a New York City attorney and two AIDS specialists from the San Francisco General Hospital Medical Center observed in a special report on infection control and public health law that ran in the *New England Journal of Medicine*.

> Balancing these interests in the context of AIDS is particularly difficult because the interests on each side are so fundamental and so strongly affected by the nature of the infection. For the individual, measures to control the spread of AIDS may invade privacy, constrain sexual conduct and procreation, and limit liberty. For the public, AIDS retrovirus infection continues to spread, especially among high-risk groups, and is often fatal; no vaccine or chemotherapeutic agent has been proved to prevent infection, reduce infectivity, or ameliorate the disease. We therefore believe that AIDS poses the most profound issues of constitutional law and public health since the Supreme Court approved compulsory immunization in 1905.[10]

In some instances, it seems logical to assume that a degree of infringement on civil liberties is justified for the greater good of the community. It is quite often the price society must pay to preserve itself against a real or potential threat. The military's decision to test its active servicemen and hundreds of thousands of applicants is one example. In that case, critics argue that the armed forces merely want to weed out homosexuals, or dodge having to provide costly and extensive medical care for those who might come down with AIDS, or both. That argument seems a bit too simple. While it is true that homosexuals do not exactly fit the military's macho image of itself, and that most commanders would not be displeased if every one of them left the service, it is difficult to fault the Pentagon for wishing to ensure the readiness and the health of its forces, particularly with regard to emergency blood donations.

Also, a compromised immune system does, indeed, leave a person susceptible to a host of other infections, particularly parasitic ones that could be contracted during overseas assignments in the tropics and in undeveloped areas, and it could trigger incapacitating reactions in personnel who require a multitude of immunizations. Military ships and barracks, like prisons and monasteries, are relatively isolated, male-dominated environments, and given the sexual needs and behavior of men in such exclusive settings, the military's order is pragmatic, if unpopular.

AIDS, once again, is a highly unusual and complex disease, one that is believed to be always fatal, and caused by a virus that, in effect, not only scoffs at the body's natural defenses but commandeers them, using them to further its own ends. Its preferred method of transmission is well known, and so, too, are its risk groups. Because of these circumstances, and if it is true, as has been suggested, that many people in high-risk groups are still donating blood despite recommendations that they voluntarily stop, management of the AIDS epidemic may, indeed, require stern measures.

Dr. Arnold Relman, editor of the prestigious *New England Journal of Medicine*, is one who has called for mandatory testing for AIDS. At a 1986 Boston meeting on the disease and public policy, Relman argued forcefully that the U.S. Constitution allows restrictions on the activities of those who are a threat to the public health, adding: "I'm not suggesting that [those who test positive] be quarantined. But it seems to me that we have to balance our concern for individual freedom and law with our concern for the general welfare." Using as an example a prostitute with antibodies to the virus, Relman concluded, "She's Typhoid Mary. Public health authorities ought to neutralize her risk to the public. They should say to her, 'You are a deadly menace to unsuspecting, uninvolved clients.' That's how I would use the test."[11]

In May 1987, President Reagan, delivering his first speech devoted solely to the AIDS outbreak, argued for widespread testing, calling for mandatory testing of federal prisoners and immigrants, and for "routine testing" of those who seek marriage licenses, a procedure that would permit applicants to refuse such tests without penalty. (Illinois and Louisiana now require testing of couples who plan to marry.) He said also that he had asked his advisers to determine whether AIDS testing might be required for those who enter Veterans Administration hospitals.

Others, however, have not been so quick to advocate such measures. Some, like the CDC's James Curran, have argued that complete mandatory testing would be difficult to implement because it would necessarily involve the enormous task of testing everyone in the United States, then doing backup tests on many of them to confirm the diagnosis. (It has been estimated that testing the 1.5 million or so individuals believed to be infected — if, indeed, they could all be identified — would cost $350 million.) Moreover, the presence of antibodies would invariably raise suspicions that a person found with them is either gay or a drug addict — characterizations that many individuals would deny, even if true. "Who out there is gay?" Curran asked an audience at an AIDS-update meeting in Washington, D.C., in 1986. "If you are, raise your hand." No one did.

"A decision to take the test must be individual, voluntary, anonymous and combined with counseling and risk reduction guidelines including safer sex practices," said a 1986 policy statement from the National Lesbian and Gay Health Foundation.

Informed consent should be a fundamental feature of any public health effort or testing program. Anyone considering the antibody test must be warned of the medical and psychological implications. Because there are now no guarantees of anonymous testing, persons at risk of AIDS also risk losing their jobs, education, insurance and right to have or rear children. The CDC acknowledges the need for anonymity in a testing program. Nevertheless, it fails to recognize [that] no state in this nation is able to offer those tested for antibodies protection from legal release of their names. Since such protection cannot be granted, all testing must be done on an anonymous basis or not at all.[12]

Such fears are well founded, but they are double-edged. For example, California and most other states, for many years, have allowed a physician to disclose a patient's infectious condition, regardless of the type of infection, to the patient's close contacts so that precautionary steps could be taken to stop spread of the disease. Recently, however, California passed a statute that forbids disclosure of the results of the AIDS-antibody test to anyone but the patient without the patient's written consent. As commendable as the change sounds, though, a conflict arises: it puts physicians in a particularly difficult situation if a patient is not taking enough care to avoid passing the disease on to others.

The authors of the aforementioned special *New England Journal* report addressed that nettling issue. After pointing out that a patient's rights mandate that doctors keep confidential all facts about diagnosis and treatment of an AIDS patient except information specifically required to be reported by a state's public health laws, the authors suggested that if a patient does not take adequate measures to avoid infecting others, doctors could directly warn any person who may be at risk (the patient's lover or spouse, for example). "Indeed, the physician has a duty to do so, but that duty would be fulfilled by reporting the patient's recalcitrance to the public health authorities, who have the responsibility for notifying contacts and other epidemiologic tasks."[13]

Apart from the danger of infecting others, a patient's recalcitrance can bring on lawsuits, criminal charges, and civil liability for damages. In several states, individuals infected with communicable diseases, such as venereal diseases, who willfully expose others to the disease, are guilty of a misdemeanor and may be fined, jailed, or both. The authors of the *New England Journal* report cite two cases. One involved a woman who claimed that she had contracted genital herpes during intercourse with a man "at a time when he knew, or in the exercise of reasonable care should have known, that he was a carrier of venereal disease" but did not disclose it. The court ruled that there was precedent for the woman's complaint, and that she could proceed at trial to prove that the facts were as she claimed. In the other pending case, a man who said he had been Rock Hudson's lover filed suit in 1985 against Hudson's estate, his former secretary, and two doctors, alleging that all parties concealed the fact that Hudson had AIDS at the time when the plaintiff and the actor were known to be sexually involved.

This difficult issue of confidentiality has also cropped up in the recent clamoring of health, accident, and life insurance companies for permission to screen applicants for new policies — a move that gay activists claim is a blatant attempt to weed out homosexuals and, thus, cut the companies' losses from AIDS deaths. The underwriters argue that if they do not obtain such permission, healthy individuals will be paying an AIDS tax in the form of higher premiums; and so they have been petitioning the states to allow questions on application forms asking whether a person is homosexual, or has been exposed to the AIDS virus, or has received a blood transfusion; some have asked that applicants be required to undergo a medical examination, including the AIDS-antibody test.

Most states allow insurance carriers to determine the health status of an applicant by the antibody test. Use of the test for this purpose is prohibited in California and the District of Columbia, and a number of other states may forbid it for insurance screening. In New York, the AIDS test is banned for hospital- and medical-insurance purposes, but is allowed for life and disability policies. Massachusetts, which originally barred the test for health, life, and disability policies, has eased the prohibition for some policies worth more than $100,000. The insurers argue that depriving them of data necessary to arrive at the probability of an event is like forcing them to drive a car while blindfolded, and submit that they have a long history of dealing with highly sensitive medical information, such as chemical dependency, alcoholism, syphilis, or a doctor's knowledge of cancer that has not been revealed to a patient. Confidentiality of results from AIDS-antibody tests, they maintain, would likewise be regarded as sensitive information, and would be protected in an equally secure fashion.

"Insurance companies need to be able to order their own AIDS-related blood tests and to use the results with all due confidentiality," says Karen Clifford of the Health Insurance Association of America.

> If insurance companies are prevented from learning adverse information that applicants already know, such unprecedented and unfair advantage will unquestionably result in attempts by people to gain from this knowledge and in consequent subsidization of those at high risk by the majority of policyholders who are at a much smaller risk of dying. Given the potential magnitude of the AIDS problem, this inequity will not only be unfair, but may well prove to have serious financial consequences to both companies and policyholders. Insurance companies must be allowed to fulfill their obligation to policyholders — an obligation that includes careful selection of applicants and actuarially sound classification practices that assure that policyholders pay a premium that is commensurate with their risk. Companies should be allowed to order their own tests, given that results will be used in a socially and fiscally responsible manner.[14]

(It should be noted here that the insurance industry once used different life-expectancy tables for blacks, and charged them higher premiums because they are more prone to hypertension and heart disease than whites. The practice is no longer permitted. There is also now a move toward "unisex rates" that would replace the current practice of setting higher rates for men because of their shorter life expectancies. In December

1986, representatives of the life and health insurance industry endorsed proposed underwriting guidelines of the National Association of Insurance Commissioners that prohibit consideration of a person's sexual orientation in the selling of insurance. But while supporting that underwriting policy, the groups urged the commissioners to amend the guidelines to permit an insurer to ask an applicant about any prior history of AIDS-related tests.)

Whether test results that signal a social disease as controversial, complex, and fearful as AIDS can truly be kept confidential is open to question. At least six states (Wisconsin, South Carolina, Colorado, Idaho, Montana, and Minnesota) already require doctors to report to public health boards not only the names and addresses of persons with a diagnosis of AIDS, but also those who test positive to the antibodies. Leaks are sure to occur in any such system.

The risks to individual rights, and the psychological consequences suffered by the person who learns he has AIDS-virus antibodies (especially when the test is conducted without consent or precounseling), are considerable; the test is not just another routine blood screening of the sort that tells someone whether the blood cholesterol level is high, or whether there is diabetes. "If we are to have any meaningful impact on the spread of this infection and its tragic consequences, counselling on safe sex and positive behavioural change must be taken into the public arena without further delay," doctors reported in April 1986 in the *British Medical Journal*. "In the present circumstances before testing doctors must ask themselves: Why are we testing and what benefits, to the individual or to society, derive uniquely from testing? How can we achieve the benefits of testing by other means? Is the potential harm resulting for the patient justified by the benefits? Do we have the means to deal with it?"[15]

Such sentiments are commendable. Education and counseling may well be better alternatives to mandatory testing, as civil libertarians and homophile groups have argued; and it is true that knowing one has antibodies to the AIDS virus does not necessarily mean a behavior change will follow automatically.

Still, there is also no guarantee that all those at high risk will seek voluntary testing, will change their behavior, or will even warn those close to them if they have tested positive. "Guidelines on safer sex must apply to all at risk," said the British journal, "irrespective of viral state. It does, after all, take two to tango, and the steps soon falter if only one partner knows the right moves."[16]

In the same issue of the *Journal*, there appears a brief article written by a gay male who tested positive for antibodies to the AIDS virus. Shocked and disoriented at the news, he woke in the mornings shaking, had trouble sleeping, lost his appetite, began to drink heavily, considered suicide, and wrote a will. Psychological counseling and a gay self-help group finally helped him get used to "being positive." He said:

> Knowing that you are positive gives you a chance to alter your lifestyle. It becomes more likely that you will adopt a healthier diet and cut down on alcohol, tobacco, or cannabis. As an actor I decided that stress was my main problem, and I took up yoga for the first time in my life with great success. The most important question is — will knowing that you are positive alter your sexual behaviour? Gays in this country have up until now followed a free and easy existence. All we risked living in the "fast lane" was, it seemed, the occasional social disease. Clearly we must adopt a more responsible attitude, and it does seem that gay men who are discovered to be positive and who are properly counselled do behave responsibly and change their sexual practices. . . . While in a perfect world all gay men should for the last two years have adopted safer sexual practices, including the use of condoms, this is not a perfect world and they have not. The reality is that at one o'clock in the morning after four or five pints in a gay pub or club gay men go home with each other without checking that one of them has condoms. I do not advocate the compulsory testing of gay men. But so long as we understand the test and its limitations and so long as good counselling is available I think we should be encouraged to take the test, both for our own good and that of the community, gay and straight.[17]

Notes

2. WHAT ARE THE SYMPTOMS?

1. "Shingles Could Herald AIDS in High Risk Individuals," news release, Society for Investigative Dermatology, 2 May 1986.
2. "CT Scan of Abdomen Helpful in Diagnosing Lymphomas in AIDS Patients," news release, San Francisco General Hospital, 25 Apr. 1986.

3. WHAT IS THE AIDS VIRUS?

1. J. Bishop, "Epidemic," *Discover*, Sept. 1982, 36.
2. J. Langone, "AIDS: The Quest for a Cure," *Discover*, Jan. 1985, 76.
3. "Patent Dispute Divides AIDS Researchers," *Science*, 8 Nov. 1985, 640.
4. "AIDS Virus Gets New Name amid Feuding," *Medical World News*, 26 May 1986, 14.
5. Ibid.
6. L. Altman, "French Sue U.S. over AIDS Virus Discovery," *New York Times*, 14 Dec. 1985, 1.
7. "A Different Kind of AIDS Fight," *Time*, 12 May 1986, 86.
8. M. Chase, "AIDS Dispute Is Tempest in a Test Tube in U.S. Lab," *Wall Street Journal*, 11 Apr. 1986, 20.
9. R. Gallo et al., "Frequent Detection and Isolation of Cytopathic Retroviruses (HTLV-III) from Patients with AIDS and at Risk for AIDS," *Science*, 4 May 1984, 500.
10. M. Gonda, "The Natural History of AIDS," *Natural History*, May 1986, 79.

4. WHERE DID THE VIRUS ORIGINATE?

1. Quoted in K. Warren, ed., *The Current Status and Future of Parasitology* (New York: Josiah Macy, Jr., Foundation, 1981), 6.
2. "NEPC Group Induces AIDS in Monkeys," *Harvard Medical Area Focus*, 10 Oct. 1985, 2.

5. HOW DOES THE VIRUS CAUSE INFECTION?

1. P. Jaret, "The Wars Within," *National Geographic Society Magazine*, June 1986, 702.
2. "Fact, Fear, AIDS," special report, Baylor College of Medicine (Waco, Tex.), Office of Public Affairs, Dec. 1985.
3. J. Levy et al., "Isolation of AIDS-associated Retrovirus from Cerebrospinal Fluid and Brain," *Lancet*, 14 Sept. 1985, 586–588.
4. "Brain Endothelial Cells Infected by AIDS Virus," *Science*, 25 July 1986, 418.
5. Ibid.
6. Ibid.
7. "Mechanism for AIDS Growth Described," *Harvard Medical Area Focus*, 6 Mar. 1986, 7.
8. Ibid.
9. "Hopes for an AIDS Vaccine Fading Fast," *New Scientist*, 3 July 1986, 28.
10. "Scientists Report New Mechanism by Which AIDS Virus Causes Cell Death," news release, Stanford Medical Center, 23 May 1986.
11. M. Chase, "New Virus Akin to Cause of AIDS Found," *Wall Street Journal*, 27 Mar. 1986, 28.
12. "Second AIDS Virus Said to Be Deadly," *New York Times*, 7 Nov. 1986, 8.
13. F. Clavel et al., "HIV-2 Infection Associated with AIDS," *New England Journal of Medicine*, 7 May 1987, 1180.
14. "Hopes Fading Fast" (see n. 9), 29.

6. HOW DID THE VIRUS GO FROM MONKEYS TO HUMANS?

1. R. Gallo and A. Sliski, "Origins of Human T-Lymphotropic Viruses," *Nature*, 20 Mar. 1986, 219.
2. J. Osborn, "The AIDS Epidemic: Multidisciplinary Trouble," *New England Journal of Medicine*, 20 Mar. 1986, 780.

7. HOW CONTAGIOUS IS AIDS?

1. Institute of Medicine–National Academy of Sciences, *Confronting AIDS* (Washington, D.C., 1986), 9.

2. Letter from W. Wertheimer and M. Rosenberg, *New York Times*, 22 Nov. 1986, 30.
3. *Proceedings of the International Symposium on HBV* (Paris, 8–9 Dec. 1980).
4. M. Sande, reply to Feb. 6 report on risk of HTLV-III transmission to household contacts, *New England Journal of Medicine*, 6 Feb. 1986, 381.

8. HOW EASILY IS AIDS TRANSMITTED BETWEEN MEN AND WOMEN?

1. L. Calabrese and A. Gopalakrishna, "Transmission of HTLV-III Infection from Man to Woman to Man," *New England Journal of Medicine*, 10 Apr. 1986, 987.
2. "Heterosexual AIDS Category Altered by U.S.," *New York Times*, 1 Aug. 1986, 31.
3. "Counting AIDS Cases Carefully," *New York Newsday*, 19 Aug. 1986, 62.
4. "AIDS Risk," in Letters, *Discover*, Feb. 1986, 80.
5. "AIDS and Intravenous Drug Use: The Real Heterosexual Epidemic," *British Medical Journal*, 14 Feb. 1987, 1.
6. J. Stibbe, "Heterosexual Infectivity of LAV/HTLV-III as Judged by Antibody Testing in Spouses of Seropositive Hemophiliacs," in *Proceedings of the International Conference on AIDS* (Paris, 23–25 June 1986), 122.
7. N. Padian et al., "Male-to-Female Transmission of Human Immunodeficiency Virus," *Journal of the American Medical Association* (hereafter cited as *JAMA*), 14 Aug. 1987, 788–790.
8. M. Vogt et al., "Isolation of HTLV-III from Cervical Secretions of Women at Risk for AIDS," *Lancet*, 8 Mar. 1986, 525–526; untitled news release, Massachusetts General Hospital, 6 Mar. 1986.
9. Untitled news release, San Francisco General Hospital, 7 Mar. 1986; C. Wofsy et al., "Isolation of AIDS-associated Retrovirus from Genital Secretions of Women with Antibodies to AIDS," *Lancet*, 8 Mar. 1986, 527–528.
10. S. Kant, "The Transmission of HTLV-III," *JAMA*, 11 Oct. 1985, 1901.
11. S. Schultz et al., "Female-to-Male Transmission of HTLV-III," *JAMA*, 4 Apr. 1986, 1703.
12. Ibid.
13. R. Redfield et al., "In Reply," *JAMA*, 4 Apr. 1986, 1705.
14. R. Wyckoff, "Female-to-Male Transmission of HTLV-III," *JAMA*, 4 Apr. 1986, 1705.

9. AIDS IN AFRICA AND HAITI

1. E. Gregerson, *Sexual Practices* (New York: Franklin Watts, 1983), 183.
2. Ibid.
3. B. Harden, "Uganda Battles AIDS Epidemic," *Washington Post*, 2 June 1986, 1.
4. Ibid.
5. M. Rosenbent et al., "Sexually Transmitted Diseases in Sub-Saharan Africa," *Lancet*, 19 July 1986, 500.
6. N. Padian and J. Pickering, "Female-to-Male Transmission of AIDS: A Reexamination of the African Sex Ratio of Cases," *JAMA*, 1 Aug. 1986, 590.
7. U. Linke, "AIDS in Africa," *Science*, 17 Jan. 1986, 203.
8. "AIDS Could Cause Havoc in Starving Africa," *New Scientist*, 3 July 1986, 24.
9. M. Demisse, "Drought and Famine," *World Health*, Aug.–Sept. 1986, 25.
10. S. Lyons et al., "Survival of HIV in the Common Bedbug," *Lancet*, 5 July 1986, 45.
11. W. Greenfield, "Night of the Living Dead . . . ," *JAMA*, 24 Oct. 1986, 2199.
12. T. Weil, *Haiti: A Country Study* (Washington, D.C.: American University, Feb. 1983).
13. T. Quinn et al., "AIDS in Africa: An Epidemiological Paradigm," *Science*, 21 Nov. 1986, 962.
14. Sir William Osler, "On the Educational Value of the Medical Society," as quoted in *Familiar Medical Quotations*, ed. M. B. Strauss (Boston: Little, Brown, 1968), 115.

10. THE ROLE OF COFACTORS

1. "Best Antidotes Are Education, Research and Behavior Change," news release, Stanford Medical Center, 23 Oct. 1986.
2. C. Russell, "Another Herpes Virus Identified," *Washington Post*, 23 Oct. 1986, A12.
3. R. Gallo, "Concomitant Infection with HTLV-I and HTLV-III in a Cancer Patient with T8 Lymphoproliferative Disease," *New England Journal of Medicine*, 23 Oct. 1986, 1078.
4. "Sex and Needles, Not Insects and Pigs, Spread AIDS in Florida Town," *Science*, 24 Oct. 1986, 416.
5. J. Levy and J. Ziegler, "AIDS Is an Opportunistic Infection," *Lancet*, 9 July 1983, 79.

6. R. Ueon et al., "Prostaglandin E2 Administered via Anus Causes Immunosuppression in Male but Not Female Rats," *Proceedings of the National Academy of Sciences* Apr. 1986, 2682–2683.

7. "UCSF Researchers Find Link between Psychological Stress, Changes in Immune System, and Recurrence of Disease," news release, University of California, San Francisco, 10 June 1985.

8. "AIDS Risk Tied to Earlier Infection," *Medical World News*, 27 Oct. 1986, 44.

9. Third International Conference on AIDS, Washington, D.C., 1–5 June 1987; news release, University of California at Berkeley, 4 June 1987.

10. N. Luban, "Neonatal Transmission: HTLV-III Implications," in *Proceedings of the NIH Consensus Development Conference on AIDS* (Washington, D.C., 7 July 1986), 88.

11. Institute of Medicine–National Academy of Sciences, *Confronting AIDS* (1986), 87.

12. A. Belman, "Brain Function Declines in Children with AIDS" (report presented at the annual meeting of the American Academy of Neurology, New Orleans, 26 Apr.–3 May 1986).

13. See note 10.

14. J. Robinson, "Army Finds AIDS Virus Exposure Higher for Blacks than Whites," *Boston Globe*, 27 June 1986, 3.

15. Ibid.

16. C. Russell, "Blacks and Hispanics Suffer High AIDS Rate," *Washington Post*, 24 Oct. 1986, 20.

17. H. Duvall, "AIDS Strikes Black Children at High Rate," Howard University Feature Service, 25 Oct. 1985.

18. T. Quinn, "AIDS in Africa," *Science*, 26 Nov. 1986, 960.

19. "Insects May Be Implicated in AIDS Transmission," news release, Mary Ann Liebert, Inc., 18 Dec. 1986; also in *Genetic Engineering News*, Nov.–Dec. 1986.

11. CAN AIDS BE CONQUERED?

1. "New Approach to AIDS Therapy," news release, University of California at San Francisco, 12 Dec. 1986.

2. Presented at the International Conference on AIDS, Paris, 23–25 June 1986; see also A. Fauci, "Anti-Retroviral Therapy and Immunologic Reconstitution in AIDS," (Laboratory of Immunoregulation, National Institute of Allergy and Infectious Diseases, 1986), 7, and L. Altman, "Physicians Describe Apparent Recovery of an AIDS Patient," *New York Times,* 25 June 1986, 1.

3. S. Krown, "Kaposi's Sarcoma and the Acquired Immune Defi-

ciency Syndrome, Treatment with Recombinant Interferon Alpha,"
supplement to *Cancer, Journal of the American Cancer Society*, 15
Apr. 1986, 1662–1665; N. Horowitz, "Small Subset of AIDS Patients Respond to Alpha Interferon: Alive up to 44 Months Free
of Kaposi's," *Medical Tribune*, 17 Sept. 1986, 1.

4. Ibid.
5. Ibid.
6. Fauci, "Anti-Retroviral Therapy" (see n. 2), 9.
7. Untitled news release, George Washington University, 22 July
1985.
8. "UC/San Francisco Team Says AIDS May Be an Autoimmune
Disease Triggered by the AIDS Virus," news release UCSF, 12
Dec. 1986 (which cites *Clinical Immunology and Immunopathology*, Dec. 1986).
9. Ibid.
10. Ibid.
11. "Hypothesis for New AIDS Treatment Evaluated," news release,
Yale University, 21 Feb. 1986.
12. Ibid.
13. Ibid.
14. "AIDS Patients Turn to Unproved Therapies," *Medical World
News*, 28 Apr. 1986, 62–63.
15. R. Robins, "Synthetic Antiviral Agents," *Chemical and Engineering News*, 27 Jan. 1986, 31.
16. D. Grady, "Look, Doctor, I'm Dying; Give Me the Drug," *Discover*, Aug. 1986, 80.
17. P. Zamecnik, "Inhibition of Replication and Expression of HTLV-
III in Cultured Cells by Exogenous Synthetic Oligonucleotides
Complementary to Viral RNA," *Proceedings of the National Academy of Sciences*, June 1986, 4143–4146; news release, Worcester
(Mass.) Foundation for Experimental Biology, 16 June 1986.
18. See note 15 above.
19. "Study Suggests a New Drug Can Temporarily Control Viral Infection Common in AIDS," news release, Stanford University
Medical Center, 27 Mar. 1986.
20. Grady, "Look, Doctor" (see n. 16), 81–82.
21. Ibid.
22. "Lab-made Vaccine for Hepatitis B Is Cleared by the FDA," *Wall
Street Journal*, 24 July 1986, 16.
23. M. Cimons, "Altering AIDS Virus May Lead to Vaccine," *Los
Angeles Times*, 31 July 1986, 1.

24. "Liability Issue Threatens Development of AIDS Vaccine," news release, Stanford University Medical Center, 8 July 1986.
25. Quoted in N. Hahon, ed., *Selected Papers on Virology* (Prentice-Hall).
26. J. Osborn, "The AIDS Epidemic: Multidisciplinary Trouble," *New England Journal of Medicine*, 20 Mar. 1986, 781.

12. PREVENTING AIDS

1. "AIDS and the Condom," *British Medical Journal*, 15 Nov. 1986, 1259.
2. "More Explicit Information on AIDS Prevention Called For at Stanford Symposium," Stanford University News Service, 23 Jan. 1986.
3. "Control of AIDS through Behavior Modification," news release, University of Michigan, 7 July 1986.
4. R. Bakeman, "Partners and Practices in the AIDS Era" (report presented at the annual meeting of the American Psychological Association, Washington, D.C., Aug. 1986).
5. J. Langone, "AIDS: Special Report," *Discover*, Dec. 1985, 53.
6. R. Sullivan, "Official Favors a Test Program to Curb AIDS," *New York Times*, 30 May 1986, B3.
7. "Needling AIDS," *Time*, 14 Aug. 1986, 27.
8. Institute of Medicine–National Academy of Sciences, *Confronting AIDS* (1986), 107.

13. WHEN SOMEONE HAS AIDS

1. *When a Friend Has AIDS* (New York: Chelsea Psychotherapy Associates, 1984).

14. AIDS TESTING

1. "Fact, Fear, AIDS," special report, Baylor College of Medicine, Office of Public Affairs, Dec. 1985, 1.
2. "Screening Blood: Public Health and Medical Uncertainty," special report, Hastings Center (Briarcliff Manor, N.Y.), Aug. 1985, 1.
3. News briefing during NIH Consensus Development Conference on the Impact of Routine HTLV-III Antibody Testing on Public Health, Washington, D.C., 8 July 1986.
4. "Cetus Technique Detects AIDS Virus," *Chemical and Engineering News*, 21 Apr. 1986, 8.
5. News release, Hill, Holliday, Connors, Cosmopulos, Inc., New York, 1 Apr. 1986.

6. A. Rock, "Inside the Billion-Dollar Business of Blood," *Money*, Mar. 1986, 167.
7. Letter from J. Hubbard ("AIDS in the Blood Supply"), *Wall Street Journal*, 8 Apr. 1986, 31.
8. M. Kruskall, "New Trends in Transfusion Medicine," in *Proceedings of the NIH Consensus Development Conference on the Impact of Routine HTLV-III Testing* (Washington, D.C., 8 July 1986), 83.
9. *MGH Laboratory Newsletter*, Jan. 1986, 3.
10. *New England Journal of Medicine*, 3 Apr. 1986; "Mandatory Testing for AIDS Rejected by UC/San Francisco Experts," news release, San Francisco General Hospital, 2 Apr. 1986.
11. R. Knox, "Medical Editor Calls for Mandatory AIDS Testing," *Boston Globe*, 4 Apr. 1986, 7.
12. NLGHF policy statement, 26 Mar. 1986.
13. "Mandatory Testing" (see n. 10 above).
14. K. Clifford, white paper, Health Insurance Association of America, 25 Nov. 1985, 8.
15. D. Miller et al., "HTLV-III: Should Testing Be Routine?" *British Medical Journal*, 5 Apr. 1986, 943.
16. Ibid.
17. Ibid.